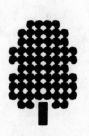

The Incredibly
LAZY PERSON'S
GUIDE *to a*

MUCH BETTER
BODY *(in Only Six Weeks)*

by Randi Blaun

LINDEN PRESS/SIMON AND SCHUSTER
1983

Exercise photographs by Sarah D. Todd

Copyright © 1983 by Randall Blaun
All rights reserved
including the right of reproduction
in whole or in part in any form
Published by Linden Press/Simon & Schuster
A Division of Simon & Schuster, Inc.
Simon & Schuster Building
Rockefeller Center
1230 Avenue of the Americas
New York, New York 10020
LINDEN PRESS/SIMON & SCHUSTER and colophon are trademarks
of Simon & Schuster, Inc.
Designed by Eve Kirch
Manufactured in the United States of America

10   9   8   7   6   5   4   3   2   1

Library of Congress Cataloging in Publication Data
Blaun, Randi.
The incredibly lazy person's guide to a much better
body (in only six weeks)
    Bibliography: p.
    1. Reducing exercises.   2. Reducing diets.
3. Exercise for women.   4. Women—Nutrition.
I. Title.   II. Title: Lazy person's guide to a much
better body (in only six weeks)
RA781.6.B58   1983   646.7′5   83-916
ISBN 0-671-47306-9
ISBN 0-671-45484-6 Pbk.

*This book is dedicated to all of you
whose sole physical activity is climbing onto and off
the bathroom scale,
and who embark on each new diet with unflagging optimism,
never giving up the dream that someday you will find a way
to have your cake, eat it . . . and not gain an ounce.*

Contents

Foreword

The first premise of *The Incredibly Lazy Person's Guide to a Much Better Body (in Only Six Weeks)* is that the reader is, sensibly, concerned about controlling her weight and about overall physical fitness; but that she thinks the time and effort demanded by the average exercise program—be it a complicated series of calisthenics or the oppressive prospect of running miles several times a week—too great a price to pay. At the same time, most women, like most doctors, now know that dieting alone is not an effective approach to weight reduction or physical fitness, and certainly not to improved health. Ms. Blaun resolves this dilemma with a program combining moderate but highly efficient physical activity with a comfortable and healthful dietary plan, which work together through sound metabolic principles to ensure weight loss and dramatic physical changes while promoting excellent health.

Many diets fail, as Ms. Blaun documents, because however great the short-term loss, they have a negative long-term effect on the body's ability to burn, or metabolize, fat. Responsible weight-control research, in which *The Incredibly Lazy Person's Guide* is thoroughly grounded, has demonstrated conclusively that unbalanced diets of the kinds promoted even in books by so-called experts are *physiologically bound* to induce a vicious cycle of weight loss and gain. Still another reason for the dieter's depression (and ultimate "failure") is that most dieters don't understand how or why any given diet is supposed to work. One of the manifold excellences of Ms. Blaun's book is that she explains correctly and simply the physiological mechanisms of weight loss, and the reasons her own guidelines will work: why, for instance, they produce only *fat* loss, as opposed to mere "weight" loss; how a diet high in complex carbohydrates can actually aid in fat removal; and why the modest amount of aerobic activity she recommends can have a dramatic positive effect on the body's ability to metabolize calories twenty-four hours a day.

Diets and even exercise programs are easily started; as anyone who has tried them knows, it is sticking to them that is difficult. But the reader of this book will discover that it is hard to fail on Ms. Blaun's plan: once motivated by knowledge, she will find the program practical, successful, and surprisingly easy.

Most readers of this book will be looking for the visibly better, more attractive body promised in the title, and they will find it. But the word "better" has more than just a cosmetic meaning here. The exercises set forth are designed not only to shape the muscles seen on the outside of the body, but also to develop and condition the muscles within—most importantly, the heart; even the reader not concerned with losing weight might consider this book a sound guide to cardiovascular fitness, which is the key to improved all-around fitness. And it would be faint praise to say of the diet presented here that it is far sounder than the average diet that promises quick weight loss. In fact, it sets forth guidelines for nutritional balance and good eating habits that any man or woman would do well to live by, year in and year out.

—Myron D. Goldberg, M.D.
Specialist in Gastroenterology
and Internal Medicine,
New York City

December 1982

1 / Six Weeks to Your Better Body—the Lazy Way

For twenty-seven years, I was lazy and out of shape.

Not that it was entirely my fault. I started out as an apparently normal infant—wiggly and voracious. But it was clear that an active life was not for me as soon as I took my first plodding, wheezing steps: I was born with exceedingly flat feet and asthma. Back then, this meant I was not only unfit to serve my country, I was to be barred from all physical exertions, specifically those that involved walking, standing and breathing.

Thus handicapped, I had to make do with the few activities left: namely, sitting, lying down and eating. Aided by an understanding and overindulgent grandmother, I managed to nibble my way satisfactorily through my formative years. With the exception of a brief, miserable stint as the most inept and lethargic goalie in the history of girls' field hockey (a position forced on me by a sadistic martinet of a gym teacher who refused to believe I could possibly have cramps three weeks out of every month), I lounged through a chocolate-covered adolescence, which prepped me for the earning of collegiate letters in snacking and snoozing. By the time I reached young deskbound adulthood, I could look back proudly on my record of never once having broken into a serious sweat.

All along, my body had been pretty decent, and forgiving of my steak-fat feasts, bonbon binges and near-total inertia. No one had yet averted his eyes in disgust as I approached, or kicked me out of bed.

But as I sauntered into my late 20s, things started to go downhill. And the same 10 pounds I had been halfheartedly trying to shed since I was a teenager had begun to look and feel like twenty.

It was time to do . . . something.

That "something" had to meet certain stringent requirements, however. It couldn't be overly strenuous or time-consuming. It mustn't demand anything so tedious as willpower, or make my stomach growl, as had so many torturous and ultimately futile diets. In short, I was looking for something that would give me the results I wanted without changing my lifestyle.

Almost as soon as my search for a painless route to a better body began, I found the first shortcuts practically at my doorstep—in the medical literature I was already consulting for various writing projects in health. I discovered that it was, in fact, the best time in history to be both vain and lazy: most of the preliminary work had already most conveniently been done for me by others.

There were the many fitness converts who had been obligingly oversweating, and the far vaster hordes of dieters who had been misguidedly undereating—both in arduous attempts to get svelte. And there were the researchers in weight control, fitness and nutrition, who used the raw material provided by these tired and hungry martyrs in an attempt to figure out just what works and what doesn't in the pursuit of a better body. But while there was ample food for thought here, I still had a lot of ground to cover. I pored over research studies, and talked to many experts; I then had to weed out the weight-control and fitness regimens that were effective but didn't suit my less-than-superhuman level of motivation. What I was left with was a collection of fresh scientific findings that all pointed to the same thrilling conclusion: a leaner, firmer, healthier, all-around better body could be achieved with far less exertion—and far more *food*—than I had ever thought possible.

By far the most exciting revelation to me was that there is actually one type of nonstrenuous physical activity—well within even my limited capacities—that could not only accomplish the longed-for reduction of excess fat from all over my body, but actually *prevent fat from forming* so easily in the future. (What was especially gratifying was how little of it I could get away with and still reap all the benefits!) I had also discovered the quickest and most efficient method of turning flab into taut flesh (a method that, unlike floor exercises, was painless and even *fun*) and trim inches off all the wrong places (such as my waistline) as well as adding them to the right ones (such as my bustline).

Naturally, I was also thrilled to learn that dieting alone is the worst possible way to lose the right kind of weight and keep it off. In fact, I was being encouraged to eat a lot *more* of my most beloved foods because they had been shown to actually aid fat loss while keeping me happily full, and to discourage fat from coming back—ever.

My final task was to put all this together in some sort of comprehensive "body renovation" plan—and put the plan to work on my body.

The result? I'm as lazy as ever, but I'm no longer out of shape. At age 33, I have a shapelier, leaner, all-around better body than I have ever had in my life.

Better means smooth curves sloping down the front of once flabby, dimpled thighs—now flaunted proudly in shorts.

Better means arms that have shed their fatty shoulder pads and underhangs.

Better means breasts that had begun what I thought was their inevitable descent toward my navel, but now stand firm.

Better means a flatter stomach and a trimmer derrière.

Better means the loss of 10 pounds of solid fat, replaced by slim, lean muscle.

And *better* means I stay slim much more easily, because my metabolism burns calories faster than ever before.

Best of all, despite years of immobility, I was able to achieve my better body with far less effort than I had ever dreamed possible.

And you can too.

The diet and exercise plans we've both tried in the past failed us because the vast majority were based on wishful thinking—not sound biological truths. Now you can finally follow a safe and nearly slothproof plan for making your body look and feel better than ever—with the rock-bottom minimum of time and effort and without hunger pangs. It's a plan whose techniques have been proved by the experts to be the most effective and healthiest of all for both modest and major weight reduction. It's a plan I know works. And if it works for me—a dedicated layabout and food lover—it can work for you. It took me twenty-seven years to find my way to a better body. But since you'll be using the shortcuts I've discovered, it's going to take you only six weeks.

A BETTER BODY—THROUGH AND THROUGH

On The Lazy Person's Six-Week Better Body Plan, you will undergo a profound physical transformation that will begin to trim off all your excess fat and literally reshape your body from your top to your bottom. And it will do this—as well as help you stay virtually fat-free forever—by correcting the biological "mistakes" that got you fat in the first place and putting your body's natural fat-burning mechanisms into action.

The Plan consists of three parts:

1. Fat-Burning Sessions
2. The Better Body Diet
3. The Better Body Shapers

The Fat-Burning Sessions—the key body-changing element of the plan—consist of a simple, nonexhausting aerobic activity you choose from among three which are specially suited for lazy persons. The Better Body Shapers, super light weight-lifting exercises, are optional: you do only the ones you feel you need, if any. Designed to firm and trim your "problem" areas, they are far less strenuous—and far more effective—than any "toning" exercises you may have tried before. The Better Body Diet rounds out the Plan. It provides sensible, nutritionally sound guidelines that let you eat far more luxuriously—and far *more*—than you ever thought possible while losing weight.

These elements work together as a team to produce a better body for you head to toe, inside and out. Why does the Plan work where diets alone (and fad exercise regimens) have failed? One, because the Plan cooperates with the physiological laws of your body which evolved over hundreds of thousands of years. Two, because it can easily fit into your current busy schedule, whether you work in an office or at home. Your Fat-Burning Sessions require a total of only two hours a week of your time, and can be done indoors, even while you're watching TV. The Better Body Shapers each take only 2–3 minutes to do—*at most*. And many can be done sitting or even lying on your bed or sofa.

Before we go any further, you should know that you don't have to spend a cent more to go on the Plan, but that you may, if you choose, spend anywhere from $10 to $450 on equipment designed specifically for lazy indoor use. (The most expensive item I recommend is, however, fully tax-deductible in many cases.) But whether or not you spend any money is entirely up to you, your choice of fat-burning activity, how (or if) you do the optional Better Body Shapers and your budget. Either way, you will still reap the full benefits of the Plan.

Here's a rundown of just some of the exciting results you'll achieve on the Plan:

A minimum 10-pound weight loss

Only 10 pounds? That's a lot less than you've been promised on all those crash diets you've tried. But unfortunately, most of the weight you lost time and time again on quickie crash diets consisted mostly of water and precious lean tissues—not fat. From now on, you'll be thinking in terms of *fat* loss, not the simple "weight" loss your scale has been mistakenly reporting all these years. Your experience on the Lazy Person's Plan will very likely be the first time in your life you've ever had a substantial loss of unwanted *fat* without also harming your other body tissues. In fact, while you are losing your fat, you will actually be building a bigger supply of the very tissue your body needs to improve and maintain its future fat-burning ability.

Since everyone's weight-loss pattern and metabolic (calorie-using) rate is slightly different, you may lose more than 10 pounds. This is especially true if you begin the Plan wanting to lose a little, or a lot, more than 10 pounds, or are tall, because initially you lose weight faster than someone who starts off closer to her target weight. In that case, the Plan doesn't have to be "over" in six weeks. It is a perfectly healthful, effective and relaxed way to lose any amount of fat weight you need to. You'll find guidelines for continuing after six weeks included in each section of the Plan.

Firmer, smoother, smaller thighs

The core of your Plan—your Fat-Burning Sessions—not only helps peel layers of fat from all over your body, but simultaneously slims what for most women is the major problem area—thighs. If you want additional firming, you can do the optional but extremely effective Better Body Shapers for thighs, which can outfirm any of the tedious "spot reducers" you've ever tried. And you can do them quickly and comfortably—even while watching TV!

A flatter stomach

The Plan will help eliminate the most stubbornly protruding potbelly, not only with fat removal from the area but with two Better Body Shapers that can tighten the entire area from your rib cage to your pubic bone. And they work—fast—even if you've just had a baby.

Firmer, higher, younger-looking breasts

Yes, you *can* do something about your breasts—no matter what size and shape they are. The Better Body Shapers for breasts can lift them, define them, make them firmer and, yes, even add inches—whatever you need most.

Slimmer, sag-free upper arms

The undersides of your arms won't be curving downward anymore if you do a few Better Body Shapers for arms. The

Plan will make inches of fat disappear from your shoulder area, too.

More fat-hungry lean body tissue

One reason you currently weigh more than you want to is that part of you actually weighs *less* than it should. You have too much fat in proportion to lean muscle tissue. Muscle is what gives your body attractive contours—and muscle "eats" more fat for energy than any other tissue in your body. So the more you have, the more fat you will be able to pull out of unwanted areas, use up and keep off your body *permanently*. This doesn't mean you must become "musclebound." The Plan simply helps give you the right amount of muscle that looks, feels and works best on your particular frame—at the very same time your fat is being swept away.

A whole new metabolism that burns calories faster throughout your body—twenty-four hours a day

Your Lazy Fat-Burning Sessions have effects that reach far beyond the loss of fat weight and the reshaping of your body. Unlike any diet, the Plan actually creates a lasting elevated calorie-burning rate in almost every organ and tissue. This helps reverse the metabolic *slowdown* in your body (which has been caused in part by dieting), and makes your body use food energy the way it was designed to use it.

A filling but fat-defeating "diet"

In order to create a better body, you must feed it right. So you won't be going on the kind of crazy unbalanced starvation or crash diets you've tried in the past—because there's ample evidence that it is precisely that kind of very-low-calorie, body-stressing dieting that actually helps *guarantee* you'll stay fat. Instead, the Plan provides you with The Better Body Diet, which encourages you to eat *more* of certain foods (including such formerly forbidden items as bread, pasta, beans, potatoes and popcorn) that not only keep your appetite satisfied but *maximize* your fat loss—with only a modest reduction in calories. Best of all, it's easy to follow: once you've looked it over and absorbed its few key nutritional concepts, you'll automatically be able to eat happily for the entire six weeks without constant measuring, weighing, calorie counting or—most important—starving. And with the help of the Lifetime Body Maintenance Eating Guidelines, you'll see how you can stay slim, energetic, healthy—and *full*—forever.

A *healthier, stronger, more energetic you*

While you're getting in shape with relative ease, you'll be getting far healthier too. Your heart and lungs will become stronger. Virtually all your body cells will be better able to make instant energy rather than fat from your food—meaning you will literally have more energy for living. Your improved muscle strength and stamina will give you the zest you need to get through everyday tasks with ease. You will handle stress better, and sleep better, and even think more clearly. And all this is happening while you are losing the fat weight you've wanted to lose for so long.

Those are the basic gains the average woman can expect from The Lazy Person's Six-Week Better Body Plan. Since there is no such thing as the "average" woman, of course, I've prepared the Head-to-Toe Quiz to help you select exactly the elements of the Plan that will mean the fastest path to *your* better body. Sit in a comfy chair, and *do* try to be brutally honest with yourself. There are no "right" or "wrong" answers . . . and anyway, they're just between *us*.

THE HEAD-TO-TOE QUIZ

1. How many pounds do you think you need to lose?
   - (a) about 10 pounds
   - (b) 10–25 pounds
   - (c) 25–50 pounds
   - (d) 50 or more pounds
   - (e) just need firming up, not weight loss

2. What would you like to do about your thighs?
   - (a) make them a few inches smaller all over
   - (b) remove puckers and dimples
   - (c) firm up the inner area

3. What would you like to do about your breasts?
   - (a) make them higher, firmer
   - (b) make them bigger
   - (c) make them smaller
   - (d) nothing—they're fine

4. What would you like to do about your waistline and stomach?
   - (a) take off inches
   - (b) get rid of "roll'
   - (c) get rid of potbelly

5. What would you like to do about your arms and shoulders?
   - (a) get rid of flab underneath upper arms
   - (b) make arms slimmer all over
   - (c) broaden sloping, narrow shoulders

6. Do you often eat when you're not actually hungry?
   - (a) yes
   - (b) no

7. Do you ever start an exercise program and quit? If so, why?
   - (a) too strenuous
   - (b) too boring
   - (c) too complicated
   - (d) too ashamed of appearance in leotard and tights
   - (e) found I preferred to lie on couch and eat bonbons

8. Do you know what "nutrient density" is?
   - (a) yes
   - (b) no—and I don't care

9. Do you want to exchange bodies with
   - (a) Brooke Shields
   - (b) Jane Fonda
   - (c) Dolly Parton
   - (d) yourself, ten years ago

10. Would you like a better sex life?
    - (a) no, it couldn't be better
    - (b) a thousand times, yes

ANSWERS

1. (a) You have never been really overweight, but you always seem to have the same 10 pounds to lose. This is caused by an extremely common combination of careless eating habits (even though you do not eat much), occasional dieting and lack of fat-burning activity. You will benefit greatly from the Plan as is. Most likely, you will lose all your "weight" before six weeks are up. But not all of that weight may be fat quite yet. Be sure to continue so you get the full benefit of the Plan—including the metabolic changes you need to *stay* slim.

(b) You have a long history of dieting. You are "busy" but very *sedentary*. You are haphazardly nourished, even though you eat what you think is a lot. You need to carefully study the Better Body Diet recommendations which will help you begin to think carefully about what you put into your mouth and why.

(c) You may be a compulsive or "binge" eater, who too often uses food unwisely as an escape or a weapon. You often eat large amounts of the wrong things, primarily sweets, and often totally neglect nutrition. You may have tried repeatedly to compensate for your overindulgence by going on very-low-calorie diets. The

Plan can spell the end of this self-punishing and unhealthful cycle of starving and stuffing yourself. It helps correct the metabolic problems caused by overindulging in sweets and being sedentary that have distorted your natural appetite. It teaches you proper nutrition. And it never lets you go hungry even while it's helping you lose weight. Also, be sure to read the section in Chapter 7 on Binge Eating.

(d) Very likely you have been overweight all your life. Perhaps you grew up in an overweight family or used food as a source of comfort during childhood. You have been trapped in a cycle of gaining/starving/gaining that has always failed, has made you fatter and has made you feel like a failure. You may think there is something physically (as well as mentally) wrong with you because you can't lose weight anymore even on a meager supply of calories. It's time to stop blaming yourself. You now have a unique opportunity to finally correct the physical and metabolic problems that have been keeping you unhappy and unhealthy and overfat. Put a smile on your face: the Plan is here to help. Throughout the text you'll find special tips on achieving your goal weight no matter how many pounds you need to lose. You will also benefit from reading the sections on Fatigue and Binge Eating in Chapter 7. You must also carefully read the entire Better Body Diet chapter. It isn't just about another diet—it teaches you a satisfying way of eating that will get you slim comfortably and help you stay that way forever.

(e) If you're at your "ideal" weight, that's great—you've got a head start on a better body. But your need for general shaping up means your muscles are not in the shape they should be in—and that you are inevitably carrying a bit too much fat in proportion to the amount of muscle you do have. So you too are a prime candidate for Fat-Burning Sessions. For maximum firmness, you should also do as many Better Body Shapers as you can. Having firmer, more active muscles in general also will prevent you from getting proportionately fatter as you get older. Though you may be eating the right number of calories, you may need to improve the nutritional content of your diet. So it's very important that you read all of Chapter 5.

2.   (a) Your Fat-Burning Sessions are essential for firming thighs,
as well as for removing fat from the entire thigh area, a process
that will be greatly speeded by the Better Body Diet. That may
be all you need. You will also benefit from doing as many of the
Better Body Shapers for thighs as you can. The Total Thigh
Shaper is especially effective for general firming.

(b) You will begin to see the effects of your Fat-Burning Sessions on this particularly stubborn problem in about three
weeks. In addition, you would also be well advised to do *all* the
Better Body Shapers for thighs, because maximum muscle development is needed to better support and smooth out tissues in
these areas.

(c) Fat-Burning Sessions alone help this area a lot, but it's
very helpful to do the Better Body Shapers for the inner thigh in
Chapter 6. It's one of the only methods of fixing this area that
you can do without being an acrobat or going to a gym. And you
can even do it lying on your bed!

3.   (a) Some women have naturally higher, firmer breasts than
other women. But all breasts (except the smallest) will eventually start to nose downward unless you do something to stop
them. Breasts lie on top of the pectoral muscles. To give breasts
the continuing support they need, you *must* develop these muscles. The Breast Shapers in Chapter 6 give truly "wow" results
in a very short time. And you even feel sexier *while* you're doing
them!

(b) The Breast Shapers in Chapter 6 are the only ways short
of surgery or weight gain that you can actually make breasts
more prominent and substantial. Believe me, they *work*.

(c) For the two or three voluptuous ladies who answered this,
there is little sympathy among your peers. But you aren't all that
smug, because heavy breasts can truly be a burden. You *must* develop your pectoral muscles to support the ample amount of
breast tissue you were blessed with. If you do this, your breasts
will look much more lush and youthful than they do now, because you will be eliminating the matronly "mushiness." Just do

the Breast Shapers in the special *slimming* way described in Chapter 6.

(d) Lucky you. But "all of a sudden" they may start to droop because your pectoral muscles are quietly getting weaker without your knowing it. Why not start doing at least one of the Breast Shapers *now*—so you'll never have to see where things may end up?

4.   (a) Fat-Burning Sessions and the Better Body Diet may be all you need to accomplish this. But I recommend you do the Better Body Shapers for the waist and stomach, say, twice a week, to keep things in line.

(b) This is a common problem for those who have frequently gained and lost a lot of weight. Whatever the case, you can benefit from doing the maximum recommended numbers of both stomach and waist Better Body Shapers. You may find that your genuine *fat* loss on the Plan has also taken care of the problem for you better than any diet alone ever has before.

(c) Most women weren't meant to have a completely flat stomach. If you can't ever iron clothes on yours—so what? But the Fat-Burning Sessions and your Better Body Diet will take off much of the cushioning. The Better Body Shaper for the stomach is the best possible way to turn your pot into more of a frying pan.

5.   (a) This is a common problem that seems to occur spontaneously with age, or after a large weight loss. The problem is twofold: excess fat and a flabby triceps muscle, one of the least-used muscles in a woman's body. The solution is to start firming it up with the Better Body Shaper for triceps in Chapter 6. Fat loss will take care of the rest of the problem. You'll see results almost immediately, because fat is often lost here first.

(b) This is also a common problem because this area is a fat-storage site in women. General fat loss as well as general firming of your arms with the Better Body Shapers for triceps and shoulders will solve it.

(c) How your shoulders look can determine how your entire body looks, because narrow, scrawny shoulders can make hips and waist appear larger. The Better Body Shapers for shoulders can give you truly gorgeous, sexy shoulders whether they're currently bony or fat-covered.

6.   (a) We *all* sometimes eat when we're not hungry, because either we're bored, something smells good or, like Mount Everest, the food is *there.* But if you have a special eating problem, don't despair—the Better Body Diet is designed to keep you *full* while you lose fat. And the entire Plan works to correct the metabolic problems that have often caused you to overeat in the past and to restore your natural, healthy appetite.

(b) You're either a saint, or lying.

7.   (a) That's understandable. Many exercise programs demand a certain level of fitness before you can even *start* them. This time, you're going to start at your *own* level, and progress at your *own* speed, so you won't ever get exhausted or discouraged.

(b) Also understandable. But the Plan gives you a choice of three fat-burning activities which you can make as pleasant as you wish. You can watch TV, read or listen to music while burning off your fat. And what could be less boring than the prospect of a new body in six weeks?

(c) Some exercise programs require so much coordination and "choreography" that you'd think you were preparing to dance *Swan Lake.* Once you have grasped the basic principles behind fat burning, you won't ever have to think about what you're doing. And rest assured, nothing in this book requires any athletic skill whatsoever beyond breathing!

(d) How you look now is one of the biggest obstacles in the way of looking better. You have simply been too self-conscious to go out and jog or join a health club and reveal those parts of you that you have been trying to hide. The Plan can be conducted in complete privacy—even away from the prying eyes of your family. Once you have your better body, you can take it out in public or to any spa with pride.

(e) So did I. Think of it this way. You're going to do the *rock-bottom* amount necessary so you can afford to eat bonbons once in a while—and burn them off faster. It won't be long before you've reached the point where you can be slothful most of the time. Part of the joy of being lazy is being free of guilt. Knowing you've exerted the barest minimum effort allows you to lie there doing nothing while still retaining some self-respect.

8.　(a) Congratulations! You must have taken a nutrition course. You also must already be skinny.

(b) Well, the bad news is that you'll have to learn to care; but the good news is that nutrient density is the one and only guiding principle you'll have to learn in order to follow The Better Body Diet. Once you absorb it, you won't have to know anything else about nutrition or food. And you'll automatically begin eating in a way that will keep you slim and healthy forever.

9.　Like (a), (b) and (c), you too have a body that is yours and yours alone, and is the sum of *your* unique parts. The Plan allows you to make the best of your special endowments while improving what needs improving most. If you chose (d), you may have a surprise in store. The Plan may make you look far better than you ever looked at *any* age, especially if you have never done anything like it for yourself before.

10.　(a) Keep up the good work.

(b) No matter how many dashing suitors are taking tickets at your door, not *feeling* attractive can definitely cramp your sexual style. Knowing your body is in the best possible shape will make you feel much more comfortable, more relaxed and far less inhibited—all of which will make you infinitely sexier to yourself and to others. And you'll almost certainly want to leave the lights on more often.

The Lazy Person's Six-Week Better Body Plan is, for you, a whole new approach to weight reduction. And you'll be using some novel tools to measure your progress on the Plan. One of those tools is an exciting new "scale" that tells you things your own scale never could. (In fact, it even proves that your bathroom scale has been lying to you most of the time.) Learning what this "scale" means to you and how to use it is the first step in the making of the much better body that will soon be yours.

So lean back, get comfortable . . . and let's get started.

2 / The New Scientific "Scale" That Tells You What Your Bathroom Scale Never Could

You might as well admit it, because I know anyway. You're having an affair.

Unfortunately, it's not with a warm, witty, understanding charmer, but with a small, cold, angular sadist, the unforgiving judge of your self-esteem: your bathroom scale.

And despite the fact that it's a stormy and profoundly unsatisfying relationship, can you bear to part?

Fat chance. You've been hooked for years, ever since you hit puberty with a depressingly fleshy thud. Indeed, you can't make it through the day without at least one demoralizing tryst (several while dieting). No matter how much abuse you take, no matter how many times you suspect you're being lied to and cheated on, you come back for more.

You're not alone, of course. Each morning, in tiled torture chambers throughout the Western world, millions of masochistic females join you in performing the solemn rite of the Mass Weigh-In. Naked and trembling, you board the tiny tyrant with dread and loathing. As the small stiletto quivers beneath your feet, you pray for mercy, a broken spring . . . but the verdict is invariably a reproach for your disgusting excesses, your gluttonous sloth. An anguished chorus of moans and *mea culpas* can be heard across the continents: "My God, how could one teeny piece of pizza weight *two pounds?*"

It's time to end it all: the dependency, the suffering, the self-flagellation. I know breaking up is hard to do—I've been there. And I'm not suggesting you go cold turkey. Weighing yourself does have its place in helping you shape up.

But it's time you learned the truth about what your scale can and can't do. It is simply *not* the all-knowing and all-powerful weight-control wizard so many quickie diet plans have it cracked up to be. It is, instead, a simpleton with limited capabilities, able to impart only, ahem, gross information about the body placed upon it. Much of the time, it tells you lies. Some are tiny ones—but most are whoppers. Because weight fluctuations can occur for a variety of reasons that have *nothing to do with losing fat*—and your scale can't tell one from another.

HOW DOES YOUR SCALE FAIL YOU? LET US COUNT THE WEIGHS. . . .

You've been on the Artichoke and Farina Wonder Diet for three whole days. You feel lightheaded . . . but so much *lighter,* too. You step on the scale, and *voilà!* You've lost 5 whole pounds! Eureka, you've done it!

You've lost 5 pounds, all right. But it wasn't 5 pounds of what you wanted to lose—fat.

Unless you run a marathon every day, or are very overweight, in three days it is *physiologically impossible* for you to lose that much fat. Almost all the weight you lose in the first few days of any reduced-calorie diet is water.

"So what if I lose water?" you say. "It's still weight. I retain water, anyway. And I'm skinnier, aren't I?" Your clothes fit. You see that thrilling drop on the scale. What more do you need to know? Like most women, you are probably convinced you are waterlogged, and that that is a major contributing factor to your weight problem. Any diet that gets rid of water is therefore a godsend.

The fact is that if you're a normal healthy woman, you do *not* ordinarily retain gallons of excess water. Nor do you store much water in your fatty tissue. The large amount of water initially lost on a diet is essential body water from your lean tissues—primarily your muscles and liver—which your body must and will replace as it adjusts to continued dieting or soon after you stop dieting. Then there are the perfectly normal adjustments in the body's water balance that can make you see a gain or loss of as much as 5 pounds per day—among them a day's high fluid intake, a full colon, excessive vomiting or diarrhea, or the ubiquitous premenstrual water rentention. Since your healthy body is about 50 percent water by weight, it monitors its precious supply constantly, and will labor to conserve water if deprived of its daily requirement or forced to give up abnormal amounts of water through dieting. But your scale can't be bothered with details. All it can tell you is that you've gotten inexplicably heavier, meaning that your diet—or you—has "failed" once again.

Not only water is lost on a diet, however: part of what you dispose of is lean muscle and other vital body tissues, along with the fat. So what your scale is reporting as a wonderful weight loss is simply the shriveling of the muscles that move your arms and legs. This phenomenon, as we'll soon see, has a *devastating* negative effect on your ability to lose fat.

The arbitrary ups and downs your scale subjects you to are frustrating enough. But what about the times it tells you you're stuck at a certain weight even when you've been dieting faithfully for weeks?

This frequently happens because you hop on the scale just as some of your lost water is returning, and at that moment, weight of fat (and precious lean tissue) lost so far equals the weight of the returning water. Again, your scale can't help you out. But taking its reading as gospel, you conclude you're doomed to be forever pudgy. You may even go on a food binge out of frustration, gaining back whatever fat you did manage to lose—and often more.

Then there's the scale's cruelest deception of all: lying to you when you are successfully losing substantial amounts of fat and fat alone.

Let's say you have about 10 pounds to lose, and frustrated by dieting, you decide to give exercise a shot. You join an exercise class, or even begin jogging a few times a week for a month or two. You keep getting on the scale, and nothing is happening. Or worse, you see a weight *gain* of a pound or more. So much for exercise. It's making you fatter!

Not so. Proper exercise makes you burn off fat and *gain* lean muscle tissue (Yes, you *want* to do that!), which weighs more than fat. So while you may be working off more pounds of flab than ever before, your scale says all that sweat is for naught.

These are all prime examples of your bathroom scale's most glaring deficiency: *it cannot tell the difference between water, muscle and fat.* And your weight is far more than the sum of your more well-padded parts. What matters most is not just how many pounds you are, but what those pounds are made of.

WHEN QUALITY, NOT QUANTITY, REALLY COUNTS

As the most respected weight-control experts and exercise physiologists now know, body composition—not body weight alone—is the critical measure of what shape you're in.

Body composition is, literally, what you are composed of,

which is primarily bone, muscle and fat. Bone, constituting about 12 percent of a woman's weight, and other body components such as skin, internal organs and connective tissue can be considered the "constants" of body composition. Although the density and weight of bone can be increased with exercise (and decreased with lack of same), skeletal muscle and fat are the two variables which can be markedly adjusted to effect weight gain or loss.

Compared with the density of water, which is 1, muscle is 1.1 and fat is .9. That may not seem like a big difference, but when attached to your body, 10 pounds of compact, slim, shapely muscle are much more esthetically pleasing than 10 pounds of fat, which takes up a lot more space and doesn't have a shape of its own. That's why a slim female athlete may weigh considerably more than she looks, and may even be "overweight" according to standard height/weight charts. For reasons we'll explore later, you don't *ever* want to lose your lean muscle tissue—*which is precisely what happens when you go on any diet.* (To look really great, in fact, you may even need to add some!) Whether or not you need to lose *weight* is therefore synonymous with whether or not you need to lose *fat*, and *only* fat. To scientists, therefore, the term "over*fat*" is more meaningful than "over*weight*."

Studies to date have indicated that the average nonobese, moderately active college-age woman who is not visibly overweight is composed of about 26 percent fat by weight, with the normal range being from 22 to 28 percent. (The average college-age man carries about 15 percent fat—a sex difference which almost surely reflects a woman's fat-dependent, energy-consuming reproductive functions.) A woman who has a 26-percent body fat level is composed of roughly one-quarter fat; if she weighs 130 pounds, she is carrying 33.8 pounds of of fat. A female body fat level above 28 percent is considered overfat.

To be sure, a decrease in your body fat percentage will occur if you've lost a considerable amount of weight by drastic, prolonged or frequent dieting. But considerable amounts of skeletal muscle may have disappeared along with the fat. You therefore see a large "weight" loss on your scale—but a grim landscape of sags, ripples and puckers in your mirror. Dieting can literally turn you into a "skinny" fat person—because you may still end up with proportionately too much fat over a shrunken frame.

That won't happen to you on The Lazy Person's Six-Week Better Body Plan, because it doesn't rely solely on your scale's reports of false "weight" loss due to yet another unhealthful, lunatic diet. Instead, it helps you achieve gradual loss of fat—and fat alone—and lets you track your progress by monitoring not only your weight loss but the critical changes in your body composition that generate your body from the inside out.

THE BODY FAT RATIO SCALE

Among the most accurate methods of determining body composition is underwater, or hydrostatic, weighing. (Fat is less dense than water, and therefore floats, while muscle is denser, and sinks. The heavier you are underwater in relation to your own body weight, therefore, the leaner you are.) Facilities for underwater weighing are, however, not yet available to the average person. Instead, you will be taking advantage of an easy-to-use yet scientifically accurate method of measuring your body fat at home: The Body Fat Ratio Scale, created by Victor Katch, Professor of Physical Education and Associate Professor of Pediatric Cardiology at the University of Michigan School of Medicine; and Frank Katch, Professor and Chairman of the

Department of Exercise Science at the University of Massachusetts.

You will use the Body Fat Ratio Scale first to determine your body fat level before you start the Plan, then once a week to monitor your continuing fat loss—always more accurately than your bathroom scale alone can do. (The Body Fat Ratio Scale is most accurate for women aged 20–40. Women over age 40 or over 171 pounds should see page 161 for an alternative method of measuring body fat.)

How to Use the Body Fat Ratio Scale:

All you need is your bathroom scale (Yes, it can be a valuable ally when you learn to read it right!), a soft measuring tape, and a pencil and paper.

1. Weigh yourself (nude, of course) preferably first thing in the morning after going to the bathroom, before breakfast and well before you expect your menstrual period.
2. On the Body Fat Ratio Scale, find the number closest to your weight and record the Factor A figure next to it on a piece of paper.
3. Measure your bare waist one inch above your navel to the *nearest* half-inch. (Do not suck in your stomach, or pull tape too tight. Such "cheating" won't give you a realistic answer . . . and you won't be helping yourself get in shape by hiding from the truth!)
4. Record the number in the Factor B column under the Factor A number.
5. Add Factor A to Factor B.
6. Subtract 12.7 from the total. *The resulting number is your body fat percentage.*

For example: You weigh 141 pounds, so your Factor A number is 15.8. Your waist measures 28.5, so your Factor B is

THE BODY FAT RATIO SCALE°

Your Weight (Factor A) + Your Waist Measurement (Factor B) −
12.7 = Your Body Fat Percentage

Weight	Factor A	Waist	Factor B
90 lb.	10.1	20 in.	15.9
93 lb.	10.4	20.5 in.	16.3
96 lb.	10.8	21 in.	16.7
99 lb.	11.1	21.5 in.	17.1
102 lb.	11.4	22 in.	17.5
105 lb.	11.8	22.5 in.	17.9
108 lb.	12.1	23 in.	18.3
111 lb.	12.5	23.5 in.	18.7
114 lb.	12.8	24 in.	19.1
117 lb.	13.1	24.5 in.	19.4
120 lb.	13.5	25 in.	19.8
123 lb.	13.8	25.5 in.	20.2
126 lb.	14.1	26 in.	20.6
129 lb.	14.5	26.5 in.	21
132 lb.	14.8	27 in.	21.4
135 lb.	15.1	27.5 in.	21.8
138 lb.	15.5	28 in.	22.2
141 lb.	15.8	28.5 in.	22.6
144 lb.	16.2	29 in.	23
147 lb.	16.5	29.5 in.	23.4
150 lb.	16.8	30 in.	23.8
153 lb.	17.2	30.5 in.	24.2
156 lb.	17.5	31 in.	24.6
159 lb.	17.8	31.5 in.	25
162 lb.	18.2	32 in.	25.4
165 lb.	18.5	32.5 in.	25.8
168 lb.	18.8	33 in.	26.2
171 lb.	19.2	33.5 in.	26.6

22.6. Factor A (15.8) plus Factor B (22.6) equals 38.4; that number minus 12.7 equals 25.7—your body fat percentage.

(These measurements were in fact my own when I was hydrostatically weighed in New York City's Queens College in one of the few such tanks in the country. The results of that test were only one-tenth of a percentage point different from the results on the Scale. So even accounting for the normal variations in body proportions, the Scale's margin of error is very small.)

THE RIGHT PERCENTAGE FOR YOU

Let's say you come up with a body fat percentage of 30 . . . a not unrealistic level for a woman who is sedentary and visibly "overweight" but not obese. As mentioned before, a figure above 28 percent is considered overfat, so you obviously need to lose some fat weight.

But even if you come in at or near the "average" body fat level of 26 percent, you may still be unhappy with the way you look. That's not only because your slugabed lean muscle mass may be underdeveloped (and actually *underweight*, as we'll discuss shortly), but because *no body fat percentage is right for every woman's body*. "Average" does not necessarily mean "ideal." The Scale's measurements were taken from American college students whose eating and exercise habits may not represent what is right for their individual bodies. Arriving at the percentage of body fat that looks good on you requires knowing how much fat you can—and can't—afford to lose.

Fat is stored in two "depots," or storage sites, the first of which is called *essential* fat. Every woman is thought to be composed of no less than 12 percent essential fat by weight, which is found in your bone marrow, internal organs, cell

membranes and fatty sheath insulating nerve fibers. Essential
fat is also required for many critical metabolic functions, including production of sex hormones. Some essential fat may
also be kept in your breasts, pelvis and thighs, the amount
varying from woman to woman.

The other fat depot, *storage* fat, is also found in the abdomen and thighs as well as directly under your skin all over
your body. (In fact, 50 percent of all your body fat is subcutaneous.) In severely overweight and sedentary older people,
excess storage fat may also accumulate in and around internal
organs, such as the heart and liver, and inside arteries.

While organ-larding, artery-clogging fat is undesirable and
unhealthy, it is the excess of subcutaneous storage fat that
creates those visible lumps and bumps you are so eager to get
rid of. But you don't want to lose all your subcutaneous fat,
because a certain amount is necessary to plump up your skin,
giving your face and body smooth, young, sexy contours. You
also need *some* of this fat as a fuel reserve. Since fat is a virtually unlimited source of energy even in the visibly lean
person, however, you don't need much to have more than
enough.

So what body fat percentage is right for you?

Because of their extremely high levels of energy output,
healthy, well-fed female athletes such as marathon runners,
ballet dancers and gymnasts may have body fat levels of 15
percent (or lower) by weight, very near their essential fat
levels. Such levels are nearly impossible to achieve or maintain if you don't exercise strenuously or—at the other end of
the health spectrum—don't regularly starve yourself.

The point here is not to turn you into an athlete or an-
orexic, but to get you to a body fat level that includes your
healthy essential fat level *and* gives you a level of subcutaneous storage fat that looks attractive on your particular frame.
Physiologists think that most women should have a total body

fat level of not more than 25 percent (including essential fat), and that a sensible base level to shoot for is 20 percent. That's not an absolute. Depending on your body and build, you may look your best at 22 percent fat, or, if you have a light bone structure, even at 18 percent. All these figures allow you a safe margin of anywhere from 6 to 13 percent more fat above your 12-percent essential body fat level.

The Lazy Person's Six-Week Better Body Plan is designed to help you gradually lose 10 pounds of solid fat while preserving and even building muscle tissue. You can figure on dropping down ½–1 fat "percentage point" on The Body Fat Ratio Scale per week—equivalent to approximately 1–2 pounds of fat. For example, if you start out at 25-percent body fat and drop down five percentage points on the Scale in six weeks, you will reach a body fat level of 20 percent. (The first week of the Plan is your body's "adjustment period," and although *your* scale will say you've lost a lot of *weight*, The Body Fat Ratio Scale will reflect your true *fat* loss, which should be 2–3 pounds.)

If you are now more than 5 percentage points above the fat level you have decided you should try for, you simply need to continue the Plan longer. Remember, you're not shooting for one hard-and-fast body fat percentage. Anywhere between 18 and 25 percent may be right for you. Wait until you've lost some fat, and then let your mirror help you decide where you belong.

WHEN "BAD" NEWS IS GOOD NEWS

Of course, you are still wondering what all this means in more familiar terms: your weight. If you lose 10 pounds of fat, you should weigh 10 pounds less on your scale—right?

Not necessarily. At some point, your scale may impart

what seems to be the most unappetizing information. After, say, three weeks on the Plan, you step on the scale and see you've lost most, but not all, of the weight you expected to have lost at that point. You get depressed and feel cheated.

Here's where your Body Fat Ratio Scale comes in again. It does what your bathroom scale, with its limited intelligence, cannot do—*it proves your "weight" loss in pounds of fat.* It's that simple. And if at the same time *your* scale says you've gained or stayed the same, that means something wonderful and exciting is happening to your body: you are trading in your fat for healthy, shapely, calorie-devouring muscle!

So the Body Fat Ratio Scale can guide you successfully through The Lazy Person's Six-Week Better Body Plan by:

- Showing you precisely how "overfat" you are now . . . so you can decide how much fat you need to lose
- Getting you through times when your scale falsely says you've gained weight
- Soothing your conscience when you've been faithful to the Plan but haven't lost "weight" at all
- Bolstering your ego until your scale reports the truth—that you have lost pounds of unnecessary storage fat.
- Alerting you to profound metabolic changes taking place in your body that can prevent you from ever getting fat or flabby again!

A little realism here. I know you'll be sneaking peeks at your "real" weight, no matter what I've told you about your scale's cheating heart. You *can't* wean yourself from a life-time addiction overnight . . . or in six weeks. But if you follow the Plan carefully, using the Body Fat Ratio Scale *once a week* as your *primary* guide, you will soon be seeing proof of the continuous loss of fat—and *only* fat—from your body for the first time in your life.

3 / From Fat Factory to Fat-Burning Machine: The Metabolic Metamorphosis

The *last* thing in the world you thought you were suffering from was anorexia nervosa. But no matter how overfat you are now, the effects of dieting on your body are not all that different from those which occur in the woman who is literally starving herself to death. And worst of all, each new diet you try is *guaranteed to make you fatter* than the one before it.

HOW DIETING MAKES YOU (AND KEEPS YOU) FAT

The Lure of the Quickie is undeniably powerful. By next Friday, you can be 10 pounds lighter, a size smaller. I know—I've been seduced by a lot of diets myself over the years. I didn't care how I got the weight off, as long as it came off *fast*. Of course, I also expected it to stay off . . . and it never did. Where was the magic I'd been promised?

The truth is, there is no magic to dieting—there's just plain old body chemistry. While there is still much to be learned about all aspects of human metabolism, enough evidence has recently been gathered about the immutable biological mechanisms of dieting to indicate that no diet alone—be it all protein, all fruit or all nothing—can ever, ever give you the lean, low-fat body you want. In fact, constant dieting will actually change your body chemistry in a way that makes you fatter far more easily. In order to understand why, you should know exactly how your body scrambles to keep itself going during that period of partial or severe caloric deprivation known as The Diet.

A Little Painless Chemistry: How Your Body Uses Energy

Your body maintains its daily metabolic equilibrium by means of a simple equation: if total calories from all nutrients—proteins, carbohydrates and fats—consumed in one day equal the amount needed for basic body-tissue maintenance (met largely by protein) and energy expenditure (met by carbohydrates and fats), weight remains the same. If more calories are consumed than can be used, weight is gained—as fat.

It should follow that any dietary regimen that reduces daily caloric intake below what your body needs will cause weight to be lost, by forcing your body to call on its stored energy for survival. And stored energy means fat, right?

Yes—and a *big* No. Body fat is your body's richest and most abundant energy source, to be sure, and powers many critical cell functions that can occur only with its help. But while some fat is always being burned, your body does not and cannot live on fat alone. During an ordinary day, 50 percent or more of the fuel you burn just to stay alive (or to move around) is the sugar *glucose*. Glucose is always found in your blood, and in every cell. But some is stored—in the form of a starch called *glycogen*—not in your fat cells but in your muscles and liver.

While each pound of fat you're carrying contains 3500 calories of potential fat energy, your total glucose reserve at any moment is about 2000 calories. So your body's reserve supply of glucose is relatively limited compared with that of fat. And your body is reluctant to use up that reserve. No matter how overfat you are, your body still needs a certain quantity of carbohydrates, from which it ordinarily makes glucose, every day—especially to fuel your brain and central nervous system, which ordinarily burn *only* glucose.

When put on a reduced-calorie regimen—which is almost invariably deficient in carbohydrate calories, as well as calories from other nutrients—your body has no choice but to call on its limited emergency supply of stored glucose. It just so happens that stored glucose is—and is *supposed* to be—chemically attached to *lots* of water. When, owing to the dietary dearth of carbohydrates, your stored glucose begins to get used up, all that water goes with it. And water is *heavy.* Therefore, if your crash diet lasts three days (about how long it takes to use up your stored glucose), you'll drop a pound for the glucose and three or more pounds of water. So far, however, you've lost just a few *ounces* of fat.

And that's just the beginning. If you continue your diet after your stored glucose has run out, your body must look elsewhere for it. If you happen to be eating any (or all) protein on your diet, your body will make it out of that, because in a pinch (and a diet is a "pinch"), protein can be broken down into glucose.

But protein isn't meant to be used as a main energy source—it's mainly supposed to build and repair your tissues. So when your body faces a glucose shortage, the dietary protein that normally would have been used to maintain your muscles and make other tissues and substances will be used to feed your brain, which is, naturally, considered less expendable. Breaking protein down into glucose is hard on the kidneys and liver, and uses *lots* of water. So *much* water, in fact, that all body tissues become somewhat dehydrated by the effort—*no matter how much water you drink.* Most of the extra pounds that seem to drop off so dramatically in the first week of a high-protein or all-protein diet are in fact pounds of water your body will reabsorb the minute you start eating like a normally omnivorous human being again.

If the diet continues longer, the situation gets even worse. In the face of a glucose shortage even dietary protein can't meet, your muscles themselves not only won't get repaired, they themselves begin to be broken down into glucose. Depending on the length and severity of your diet (severe meaning very-low-cal regimens or no-protein, all-fruit diets), *from 30 to 65 percent of the weight you lose may be lean muscle tissue.* So after your "successful" three-week diet is over, you will certainly look "slimmer," weigh less and have lost *some* fat—but at what cost? You could have lost the same 20 pounds simply by cutting off your leg.

Losing muscle (and other lean, protein-containing parts of yourself, such as skin and internal organs) is unappetizing, cosmetically horrid and, if taken to the extreme, even life-threatening. And it is also self-defeating. Why? You may not care about losing your muscles, as long as you look slim. But it is this phenomenon which dooms every diet, and your chances of *staying* slim. Losing your lean muscle tissue enhances your potential to get fat again by ruining your ability to burn the fat you have and guaranteeing that the calories you eat in the future will turn into even *more* body fat.

While your fat tissue is incredibly "lazy," usually occupied between naps mostly with making more of itself, muscle is designed to keep busy building and repairing itself, and doing everything from carrying your luggage to allowing you to yawn. All this burns calories of body fat along with glucose.

So it follows that the less muscle you have—and you have less and less each time you diet—the harder it is to use up calories and burn off your stored fat.

The processes just described happen to a lesser or greater extent on all diets. But fad diets not only take advantage of these irrevocable metabolic events, but manipulate other physiological systems as well, making it seem that you're losing more, faster, than ever. Protein diets are so popular because they seem to make you lose weight speedily—but that loss is mostly water which is bound to come back. An all-fruit diet will really go to town on your muscles and other tissues, because there's no protein at all to maintain them; any *very*-low-calorie diet (liquid or solid) will digest that much more of those tissues. Fasting is utterly ridiculous, for reasons that should be obvious by now. (When nothing is coming in, your body literally has nothing to eat but itself—and most of the self eaten initially isn't fat.) And—sorry—all the diet pills in the world can't change these facts.

Of course, as veteran dieters know, if you can starve yourself for more than three weeks, your body does begin to adapt to dieting. If the diet is at least a balanced one, including minimum amounts of protein and carbohydrates, lean-tissue loss decreases, and fat begins to be called on to supply more and more of the body's energy requirements usually supplied by carbohydrates. Even your brain may begin to use some fat by-products called ketones (this state is called "ketosis," which is often accompanied by a feeling of lightheadedness or dizziness). But it takes at least three weeks to begin to lose substantial poundage from where you *want* to lose it—your under-skin fat tissue. Since most popular diets—by design or desire—don't last that long, you are soon back where you started—overfat—and have put the rest of your body through the wringer to boot. You've lost much of your precious fat-burning equipment—your muscles. And your crazy fad diet has taught you absolutely *nothing* about how to eat happily and well to get and stay slim.

Of course, a nutritionally balanced diet and *modest* reduction in calories does have its place in your achievement of a permanently lean and better body and is, therefore, part of the Plan. But the one principle you *must* grasp is that no diet—no matter how "healthful"—can by itself remove fat and fat alone and, most importantly, keep you lean forever.

Getting Fat on Half the Food

By repeated dieting, not only do you keep losing more of the engines that burn fat, *you are increasing your entire body's ability to conserve fat and make more fat!* Even a brief crash diet can alter body chemistry enough to cause enhanced storage of fat not only on the diet but for months afterward.

How does this happen? Deprived of its accustomed ideal maintenance dose of calories, your body becomes downright stingy with energy expenditure. Within a few days—or within hours if you are fasting—your body begins to turn down your *basal metabolic rate* (BMR), which is the rate at which calories are consumed by all body systems when you're at rest. Fewer calories become available for such optional quick-energy activities as climbing stairs (or even standing up), because calories must be carefully apportioned to keep your brain and vital organs going. Depending on the length and severity of caloric restriction, your BMR may drop anywhere from 10 to 50 percent! The end result is that you may adapt to living, however listlessly, on as few as half the calories you did before.

Naturally, that means less fat will get burned. But worse yet, while you seem to be getting "skinnier" and you may be losing "weight," your body is secretly becoming much more efficient at manufacturing fat! Your diet has made your body think it can't rely on a regular "maintenance" food supply, and when sufficient food is available again—which is to say, when you end your diet, or binge out of perfectly understandable hunger—it will eagerly snatch up a higher proportion of calories and hoard them as body fat than it would normally have done before you dieted. *That's* why you gain weight back so fast after dieting even when you aren't overeating, but are simply consuming what would formerly have been your "maintenance" level of calories. And don't forget, your metabolic rate has been lowered, meaning your whole body will *continue* to burn fewer calories than you did before dieting. So, after gaining back your old pounds—and probably more—you find you must go on another, even more severe diet, and make your metabolism even more energy-conservative and fat-producing. Coupled with the loss of lean, energy-devouring muscle tissue that invariably accompanies dieting, this process has made you into a fat factory. And the fatter you are, the more efficient is that factory.

Survival of the Fattest

Perhaps you have concluded that your body is hopelessly stupid. You deprive it of food, and instead of using all that extra energy you've socked away, it jealously guards your fat supply and downshifts your metabolism so that even more fat is made out of the meager calories you *are* consuming.

There's a method to this seeming metabolic madness. While you are concerned solely with the cosmetic benefits of purging your fat cells, your body has been programmed to care about one thing: survival. Fat is a rich, powerful and precious fuel which is critical to many life-support systems, and can maintain the body through a prolonged period of caloric deprivation. Having a goodly supply of fat is like having a gas tank that's always full—and no doubt gave our ancestors (who, it must be remembered, did not "diet" by choice) a definite survival advantage during droughts, famines and illnesses. Since women had to have sufficient energy reserves to get through the energy-demanding tasks of pregnancy and lactation, we became especially adept at fat-making.

By frequent dieting, you are subjecting your body to periods of semistarvation far more often than was ever likely to happen in nature. You are unwittingly putting into operation mechanisms that evolved to keep you alive until the next meal wandered by. Since your body can't tell the difference between starvation and self-improvement, it concludes it's living in a calorically unreliable environment and therefore behaves conservatively, keeping you as fat as possible and quickly helping you store *more* fat when food *is* available again before the next cosmetic "famine."

Fitting into Your Genes

If that were the end of the story, you and I and every other sometime dieter would be forever fat. But while your body fights hard to prevent you from wasting away to nothing, evolution didn't declare that you must be permanently pudgy, either. By calling on yet another ancient genetic capacity, you can transform your metabolism and your body from a fat maker into the fat consumer it was meant to be—and even undo the damage done by dieting.

YOUR FAT-BURNING ENGINES—AND HOW THEY (SHOULD) RUN

Despite a more-than-adequate diet, it is unlikely that early humans ever became obese or even pleasantly plump, since the hunting and gathering of food as well as the general tasks of living kept everyone busy most of the day. Just in the last century, however, we have altered our lifestyles dramatically. We don't hunt, we don't dig, we don't plow. We live our lives in chairs. This has disrupted the critical energy equilibrium between caloric intake and energy output that the human body was designed to maintain.

What this means is that you have inherited a body that is *supposed* to eat well—even heartily!—and then constantly use up calories by moving around a lot. Continuous movement of muscle—especially the leg muscles—burns a lot more calories than anything else your body can do.

Not moving muscles regularly, therefore, is unnatural, and throws every body organ out of whack and into a fattening nap. What's more, inactive muscles make your entire body look saggy, whether you're very or even just a little overfat. Fat has almost no shape of its own, relying almost totally on the underlying muscles to give it attractive contours. So a firm body is a body with good muscle tone—whether that body is male or female. But muscles don't spontaneously stay firm: it's a case of use 'em or lose 'em. Luck of the genetic draw may have endowed you with a tight skin "wrapper" that keeps you *looking* firm for years—the blessing of youth. Then "all of a sudden" everything takes a trip south. As the years whiz by, all those underused muscles are quietly shrinking, meaning that even if you maintain the same *weight* from ages 25 to 40, that weight is composed more and more of *fat. Muscle cannot turn into fat.* What happens is that fat cells get fatter, and the muscle cells get thinner.

What is the solution? Obviously, *some* form of regular physical activity—meaning the movement of muscles—is *absolutely, positively essential* to the creation of a permanently leaner, energy-burning, better body. Only your muscle cells are capable of gobbling up really huge amounts of the body fat you have too much of, and getting you down to the pretty, sexy, individually *right* body fat level you were meant to have in the first place.

"Uh-oh," you're thinking, "here come the wind sprints and the push-ups. This isn't a book for lazy people after all!"

Rest assured, the biological facts and I remain true to the title's promise, because the kind of physical activity that makes you instantly purple in the face and half-dead from exhaustion is precisely the kind that does *not* use up your body fat most efficiently.

Sugar Power . . .

There are basically two ways a muscle can be moved—and each requires its own special "energy food."

When you must exert sudden or maximum muscular effort, such as sprinting for a bus, lifting a very heavy weight or even doing a very fast set of calisthenics, your muscles use mostly calories of glucose for energy. This process of energy production is called *anaerobic*, meaning "without air," or oxygen, because glucose doesn't have to have an immediate supply of oxygen to release its energy. Instead, it can break down by itself, and the by-products wait for oxygen to show up later to help form waste products—completing the cycle of energy release. (This is why you pant so hard after running for that bus: you are paying back that "oxygen debt.")

While glucose comes in very handy for quick or very intense bursts of muscle effort, you can't continue that kind of effort for long. The tiny glucose "tanks" in the muscles being used are soon emptied, and you poop out. Before you can again perform any kind of intense physical activity with that particular muscle group, you have to wait until carbohydrates you've eaten refill them with glucose. (A special kind of anaerobic activity does have its place in the making of a better body. It is what you'll be doing if you do any of the

Better Body Shapers, which have a unique talent for quickly firming up parts of you that have until now remained stubbornly flabby and resistant to exercises.) So anaerobic muscle activity isn't the ideal way to burn many calories, because you don't do it for long. And even the calories you do burn aren't calories of your body fat.

... and Fat Power!

When you are not dashing for a bus or doing jumping jacks, but are simply engaged in all the humdrum biological tasks of staying alive, you receive your caloric energy from a mixture of glucose and fat. This team-effort release of energy, which provides caloric "juice" to all cells—including muscles—requires a steady supply of oxygen, which you are always obligingly inhaling just for that purpose. It is therefore called aerobic ("air-using") energy production.

While you are typing, or just lying there reading this book, you are, therefore, operating on aerobic, fat-burning energy—though at a *very* low level.

But when you call on your muscles to move at a steady—but not blistering—pace for more than a few minutes, truly terrific things begin to happen to your fat cells.

Vacuuming Your Fat Away

Your body knows it can keep going almost indefinitely on the virtually unlimited supply of energy that is stored in your body fat. So when it realizes that you're asking just for a moderate level of continuous movement rather than heavy, or quickly tiring, effort, it obligingly shifts metabolic gears, stepping up your normal aerobic energy production from low to high.

That's when fat begins to burn. At first, more glucose is

used than fat. But after just a few minutes of moderate but continuous movement go by, the muscles get hungrier for fat than they do for glucose. To satisfy their growing appetite, a steady stream of fatty acids begins pouring out of fat cells *all over your body.* That means fat is "vacuumed" out of your thighs, abdomen, derrière, hips, upper arms—anywhere you have extra fat stored—and whisked to the moving muscles to be set on fire and lost *forever!*

It is this kind of aerobic, fat-burning muscle activity that is the key to your better body—not only because it empties your fat cells, but because, as we'll discuss shortly, it sets your body's metabolic rate higher in general, so that you are burning fat faster than ever before *all* the time, even while you sleep. And a faster metabolic rate means that calories you eat in the future aren't nearly as likely to end up as fat. Your whole body literally turns into a perpetual fat-burning machine!

The best news is that putting this powerful natural fat-removal system into action isn't hard at all. Allowing your muscles to be the fat-burning engines they were meant to be (and if need be, better fat "sculptors") is actually quite pleasant. You simply have to give them enough of a periodic "overload," which is simply anything somewhat more strenuous than the muscle is accustomed to. And you do that with Fat-Burning Sessions and, if you wish, with Better Body Shapers.

A FINAL GOODBYE TO ALL THAT FAT—THE LAZY WAY!

Awakening sleeping muscles and switching on a long-dormant metabolism doesn't happen overnight. But you'll be amazed at how eagerly your body responds to gentle and gradual encouragement. A simple formula lets you adjust your Fat-Burning Sessions precisely for your age and current condition, so that you are always doing just enough to continuously improve your fat-burning ability, *but never enough to exhaust you.* It should be obvious that to do fat burning successfully, you don't have to be a marathon runner. You don't have to be the least bit athletic or even be particularly coordinated. Even the laziest of bodies can begin the transformation from fat factory to fat-burning machine in only six weeks.

A better body, of course, isn't just a busier body—it's a well-nourished body. It shouldn't be a hungry body. By absorbing the few simple nutritional concepts and following the eating plan presented in Chapter 5—The Better Body Diet—you will be eating better (and probably a lot more) than you've ever eaten on a diet, while steadily losing all the fat weight you need to lose.

On top of it all, you'll be rewarded with a healthier heart, stronger bones and joints, more energy, reduced stress and tension and even more radiant and younger-looking skin!

And now, The Lazy Person's Six-Week Better Body Plan.

4 / Fat-Burning Sessions

The Plan is designed to make major internal and external changes in your body and produce a 10-pound fat loss in just a few short weeks. The key to all these things is your Fat-Burning Sessions. They guarantee you'll lose fat fast. And they change your body not just cosmetically, but *chemically*, so you'll be able to keep your better, leaner body once you've got it.

The Plan gives you a choice of three fat-burning activities which have been selected specifically for lazy—and busy—people and tailored so they can fit neatly into anyone's schedule. You will be doing four 30-minute Sessions of your chosen activity per week, which a survey of major clinical weight-control programs has indicated is the rock-bottom minimum requirement for speedy and successful fat removal.

YOUR PERSONAL FAT-BURNING HEART RATE RANGE

There's only one item you need to keep track of other than time and frequency of your Fat-Burning Sessions, and that's your heart, or pulse, rate. Your heart directs the entire aerobic operation, as it is responsible for pumping more and more oxygen-rich blood from your lungs to your working muscles so that they can in turn ignite more of your fat. Your heart rate per minute therefore tells you whether you are performing the correct intensity of continuous muscle movement to call on stored fat for fuel. Thus, you will periodically be checking your pulse rate at certain points in your Session.

How to Take Your Pulse

Taking your pulse is easy. Just place the first two fingers of one hand on the side of your neck under your jaw. You will find an indentation where you will clearly feel the throbbing of your carotid artery. (Do not use your thumb, because it has a pulse of its own.) Using a watch with a second hand, or a digital watch, count the beats for 10 seconds. Multiply that number by 6. That is your pulse rate per minute.

Calculating Your Fat-Burning Heart Rate Range

The ideal fat-burning state is achieved at a heart rate that falls anywhere between 70 and 85 percent of the *maximum* heart rate possible (during all-out effort) predicted for your age. From a teenage high of about 200, maximum heart rate declines about a beat per year after you reach about age 20. A good formula for calculating your current maximum heart rate is:

$$220 - \text{Your Age} = \text{Your Maximum Heart Rate}$$

If you are presently 32 years old, your maximum heart rate is 220 minus 32, which is 188.

This is *not* the heart rate per minute you will need to achieve during your Fat-Burning Sessions! Maximum or near-maximum heart rates are achieved only during quick anaerobic exercise, such as sprinting, and can't, of course, be kept up for long.

Instead, you will be working within your Personal Fat-

Burning Heart Rate Range, which is any rate that falls between 70 and 85 percent of your maximum heart rate. The 70-percent level can be considered your "threshold," or Base Fat-Burning Rate—just stimulating enough to switch on and continuously improve your fat-burning capacity, but low enough so that you can sustain the activity for more than a few minutes. Your body will, of course, feel as if it's doing some work—but you will not, and should not, at any time feel so exhausted that you can't continue.

Your breathing rate will, of course, also be somewhat elevated, but you shouldn't be panting. In fact, some physiologists call fat-burning activity "conversational exercise," because you should never get so breathless that you can't carry on a conversation while you're doing it.

The formula for determining your Base Fat-Burning Heart Rate is as follows:

Your Maximum Heart Rate × .70 = Your Base Fat-Burning Heart Rate

So if you are 32, and your maximum heart rate is 188, your Base Fat-Burning Rate is figured as follows: 188 × .70 = 131.6. If you come up with a number like this, round it off to the next highest number, which is 132.

The last figure you need to calculate is your Top Fat-Burning Heart Rate, which is the highest rate at which you should *ever* attempt to exercise. (It isn't necessary—or advisable, at least at first—to exercise at this rate, but it gives you a "ceiling" for your Fat-Burning Session.)

Your Top Fat-Burning Heart Rate is figured in the same way:

Your Maximum Heart Rate × .85 = Your Top Fat-Burning Heart Rate

At 32, your maximum heart rate is 188; 188 × .85 = 159.8—which rounds off to 160.

So if you are 32, your Personal Fat-Burning Heart Rate Range is 132–160 per minute. During your Fat-Burning Session, any heart rate you reach *within* that range that you can comfortably sustain for the entire Session will ensure that you are burning off your body fat.

Depending on the fat-burning activity you've chosen, it will take from 3 to 10 minutes for your heart to warm up to your Base Fat-Burning Heart Rate or beyond. Once you reach that rate, you must then do a minimum of 20 minutes of fat-burning activity at that rate. I've tailored your Fat-Burning Sessions so that no matter which of the three activities you choose to do, you will always get at least the essential *minimum* of 20 minutes of fat burning within a 30-minute Fat-Burning Session.

To see if you are at your correct Fat-Burning Heart Rate, pause briefly and take your pulse 10 minutes into the Session, by which time you should have warmed up to your correct pulse rate regardless of the activity you've chosen. If your pulse is too low, you can increase the intensity of your Session. If it is too high, you can decrease the intensity. As a double check you can also take your pulse immediately— within 10 seconds—after the Session is over.

After a few Fat-Burning Sessions, you may no longer need to take your pulse because your body will be able to sense whether you are working too hard or not hard enough. Be sure to check your pulse while exercising at least twice a week, however, because you want to guarantee that your Fat-Burning Session is doing just that—burning fat.

Checking Your Progress

In the first two weeks of your Plan, it may not take much effort on your part to reach your 70-percent Base Fat-Burning Heart Rate. As the Plan continues, your heart and muscles will begin to get into such good, strong condition they will have to exert less and less effort to do the same amount of work. Your body is becoming more efficient at burning fat. So you can expect to increase the intensity of your Fat-Burning Session periodically to stay at your 70-percent level and to experience further fat-burning and conditioning benefits.

The higher you push your heart rate within your Fat-Burning Range, the more calories you will burn. But for the first two weeks, you should work at or near your Base Fat-Burning Heart Rate. You *must not* rush things. If you push your heart rate too high within your Fat-Burning Range during the first two weeks of your Plan, you will tire easily. After two weeks, you may want to try to do your Session (or part of it) at a slightly higher heart rate—say, at your 75–80-percent level—or do a longer Session—say, 45 minutes—once a week. I feel most comfortable these days working at the upper end of my Fat-Burning Range, at about 80 percent of my maximum heart rate, and I often pedal 45 minutes to an hour. But if on some days I'm feeling less energetic, I simply stay at my 70-percent level and do 30 minutes. Just do what feels good for you. Remember, you don't ever have to do your Sessions at higher than your 70-percent level to continue to burn fat and to experience all the important metabolic changes that come with fat burning.

Special Note: If you haven't walked more than a few blocks for twenty years, or are very overweight, you should start at 50–60 percent of your maximum heart rate, then *slowly* build up to 70 percent or higher when you feel you're in better condition. The worse shape you're in now, the faster you'll feel and see the improvements in your stamina and muscle tone. Of course, if you have a history of heart or artery disease, high blood pressure, diabetes or any chronic disorder, you should consult your physician before engaging in any unaccustomed physical activity.

HOW, WHEN, WHERE: FITTING YOUR SESSIONS IN

Because you lead a busy life, you may be wondering just how you can find the time for *one* Session, much less four. Between your job, the kids, the house, your friends and your spouse, you haven't a minute to yourself.

Well, everybody's busy these days. It's a question of priorities: if you put your personal well-being at the bottom of your list—somewhere below washing the dog—you will always neglect it. You wouldn't think of going without brushing your teeth or bathing. You must come to consider your Sessions equally important. Fat burning isn't merely a bit of cosmetic self-indulgence: it's a serious attempt at improving the state of your general health.

Since we do tend to live by the clock, it's especially handy that your Sessions come in neat half-hour packages that allow you to plug them in at any time during the day. Two of the fat-burning activities are done indoors, and during both you can easily watch TV or listen to music. One even lets you read or talk on the phone while you do it!

The time of day you do your Session is up to you. You can do it when you get out of bed in the morning (I am not what you'd call a "morning person," but I find that moving muscles is a nicer way to wake myself up than an alarm clock), or you can wait until after having a light breakfast. Then you can hop into the shower or tub.

If you are a night owl, you can do your Session during the news, or later after dinner; it's a great sleeping pill. (Some people find they get too revved up to sleep if they do a Session right before bed, however. See how it feels for you.)

There are many ways to wedge your Sessions into even the busiest day. You can do them during lunch at work, or during your baby's nap. You can make an appointment with yourself always to do one during a child's Scout meeting, or just before your spouse comes home from work, or while dinner is in the oven. Your pattern of Sessions can vary from week to week, or you may feel more comfortable setting a regular time. Do them all in a row . . . every other day . . . whenever they fit your schedule and your mood. It's up to you. You may find it helpful to check off your Sessions on a large wall calendar.

THE CALORIE COUNTDOWN

The fat-burning activities you'll be doing will help you burn *approximately* 8 calories per minute once you reach and stay at your Base Fat-Burning Heart Rate and about 10 calories per minute if you ever decide to work at the upper end of your Fat-Burning Range: in other words, 240–300 calories per Session. On top of that, your body will use at least another 50 or so calories after your Session just returning itself to a resting state—for a total caloric "cost" of 290–350 per Session, or 1160–1400 calories per week. But caloric expenditure during your Sessions is not as important as the chemical changes that make your whole body use calories faster than ever before as a result of your Sessions. The general boosting of your metabolic rate will keep your body burning fat faster twenty-four hours a day, seven days a week. You will literally get slimmer while you sleep.

And while all these transformations are happening, by the way, the one muscle that is *really* responsible is quietly shaping up inside: your heart. Having a strong heart (and lungs) may not be your prime concern, but it's a welcome bonus of fat burning. A strong heart can pump more blood per beat than a weak one, and therefore doesn't have to beat as many times in a minute—or in a lifetime—to do the same job. (You may, in fact, notice that after a few weeks on the Plan, your resting pulse rate drops by as much as 20 beats per minute!) A stronger heart can handle physical or emotional stress better, and recover faster. A stronger heart is less likely to have a heart attack—and more likely to recover from one. You can't see it in the mirror, but a stronger cardiac muscle is literally the heart of a better body.

THE LAZY PERSON'S FAT BURNERS

To qualify as a fat burner, an activity must involve the *continuous, rhythmic* movement of muscles. While any muscle can theoretically perform aerobic fat-burning work, the larger the muscle (or muscle group), the more energy and oxygen it requires when it moves. Large muscles are therefore best equipped to produce the elevated heart and breathing rates essential to the fat-burning process. A fat-burning activity is one that almost always calls primarily upon the biggest muscle groups in the body, which are in the legs—specifically the thighs—and the buttocks.

While a fat-burning activity must be continuous, it must *not* wipe you out. I can't stress this enough, since so many people are convinced that the only kind of exercise that will make them lose weight is one that makes them half-dead and causes pain. I have often seen people at health clubs swim furiously halfway across the pool, then, unable to crawl another stroke, gasp, "I'll *never* get in shape; I can't even swim *one lap.*" And I've witnessed others racing their pulses around the block only to collapse in a wheezing heap and swear off running forever.

Now hear this: it is a puritanical and stubborn misconception that you have to *suffer* to become fit and slim and gorgeous. In fact, suffering is counterproductive, since, as you'll recall, all-out exertion *doesn't burn fat.* While doing the *right* kind of activity you do breathe a bit faster, and you should also expect to sweat a little. Fat burning (yes, the fat is literally burned) generates a lot of heat, and sweating is your body's way of cooling off. But your fat-burning activity will always be something you are able to continue to do for your entire Session *comfortably,* while being just invigorating enough to keep your pulse rate in your magic fat-burning range.

There are lots of excellent fat-burning activities around. Heading the list in popularity are running and jogging, followed by bicycling and swimming. Cross-country skiing, mountain climbing, hiking, ice skating, roller skating, jumping rope, and tap, disco and aerobic dancing are also fun and effective.

If you were doing any of these regularly, of course, you wouldn't be reading this book. At some point, perhaps at the end of the Plan, you may wish to get involved in one or more of these sports or activities on a regular basis. And in fact, the Plan will get you into the kind of shape that will help you *start* doing any activity you've always wanted to do in decent shape.

But right now there are numerous reasons besides laziness why none of the above are right for you. Some require special facilities, which are too much trouble to get to. Some make you go outside, which may not be to your taste in bad weather . . . or *any* weather. Some are initially too strenuous for someone who hasn't moved in years—or ever. Perhaps you have small children, which makes it hard to leave the house by yourself. Maybe you'd simply like to feel more secure about the state of your thighs before you take them out in public. To top it off, you are just too busy.

The whole point of the Lazy Person's Plan is, of course, to get you in very respectable shape at your convenience, with a minimum of fuss, preparation or disruption of your life. You need a fat-burning activity you can do easily, at or near home or in private, at an intensity you can control very carefully.

The Fat Burners that fill these requirements perfectly are:

1. Stationary Cycling
2. Rebound Jogging
3. Walking

The following sections will tell you all you need to know to pick the fat-burning activity that suits your needs best.

1. Stationary Cycling

Like regular biking, stationary cycling is an excellent fat burner and is an especially effective thigh tightener. But it doesn't require a road or nice weather. You don't have to leave home. You can read, watch TV, even knit while you pedal, in a blissfully climate-controlled environment. And you do it sitting down. It is, to me, the best lazy way of all to burn fat—and the one that played the major role in burning off mine.

Stationary cycling is the fat-burning activity to choose if you have small children and can't leave home. It is also the best activity if you are starting out more than 50 pounds overweight, because it prevents the stress on weak joints that excess weight can cause during a weight-bearing exercise such as jogging. It also allows you to carefully and gradually adjust the intensity of your exercise, which is difficult to do with exercises that demand a certain initial level of fitness just to do them correctly.

What to Look for in a Bike

While there are inexpensive devices for converting a regular bike into an indoor exerciser, they don't work very well.

You're much better off with a bike built for that purpose. You should also forget motorized bikes which produce *passive* pedaling or rowing motions: they are useless for fat burning or anything else.

A serious fat-burning machine first of all has some way of creating resistance against which you pedal; that's how you get your heart rate up. The best resistance mechanisms are clamplike brakes, called calipers, on either side of the wheel, or a friction belt that wraps around the wheel. (There are electronic braking devices as well, but they are found on very expensive bikes used for monitoring exercise programs for heart patients.) Roller-type brakes on top of the wheel are hard to adjust precisely and produce a jerky pedaling motion that can hurt your knees. Do *not* buy a bike that features this kind of brake.

Other essential elements of a stationary bike are: a weighted front wheel or a flywheel (a wheel with spokes is unnecessary on an indoor bike); a braking control knob or lever that permits small adjustments in braking resistance; a comfortable, adjustable seat and a speedometer and odometer. A timer is optional, but handy and motivating. The handlebars should be adjustable but not movable—rowing while you pedal doesn't help you burn fat better and may throw your back out.

I have had a Schwinn exercise bike for seven years. I have spent many happy hours biking while watching TV, reading (from the bike's reading stand) and doing crossword puzzles. I have pedaled the equivalent distance in miles from New York to California, and am currently on my way to Alaska. I give my bike almost full credit for totally revamping the lower half of my body. In just a few weeks after I began using it— and I had been virtually immobile for years—my thigh dimples began to disappear. My inner thighs firmed up. Gentle curves (not bulges) began forming where I wanted them. The legs of my pants were looser. All this happened without any weight loss, because I was simultaneously losing fat and gaining muscle.

Cancelling Your Reservations—and How to get a (Tax) Free Ride

Perhaps you balk at having a bike around the house—especially if your house isn't a house but an apartment. I live in a New York City studio. Unless I'm having a large party, I leave my bike in plain view. It's a conversation piece. If you truly want a better body, you *will* find a place for your bike. Consider it an essential appliance, as you do your refrigerator.

Then there's the price. A top-quality exercise bike—and that is the only type worth considering—costs from $225 to $450. Well, if you add up all you've spent over the years on things like sauna suits, diet pills, diet foods and fad diet books—not to mention the health-club membership you never used—you can see what a bargain you're getting. A good stationary exercise bike is *not* just another piece of faddish junk. It is a serious physical conditioner often prescribed by physicians as part of a treatment program for cardiovascular disorders, high blood pressure and diabetes, as well as for weight control—*and in these cases, it is one hundred percent tax-deductible as a medical expense.* Even if you have none of the above conditions, you may still be able to deduct the cost of your bike: if your doctor is among the increasing number of physicians who recognize that physical activity is important to your health, he or she may be willing to prescribe it for you. And long after it's paid for itself, your bike will keep on burning your fat, because a good bike lasts a lifetime. Even if you move on to other activities, it can always be used when the weather is bad. I occasionally do other fat-burning activities these days, but I still come back to my bike every winter, and when I can't go out or don't want to.

Pedaling in Comfort

You can wear anything while pedaling that's loose, comfortable and seamless. I usually wear running shorts and a T-shirt. Sweat pants are okay in winter if the room in which you pedal is very cold; otherwise you will get too hot. You can pedal barefoot, or in rubber-soled shoes, but I prefer to wear the kind of half-socks made for tennis. I also recommend placing half-socks over the grips on the handlebars to absorb sweat from your hands, and draping a small towel over the front of the bike to use on your face.

How to Use Your Bike for Successful Fat Burning

Here's how to get yourself and your bike ready for your Fat-Burning Sessions:

1. Sit on the bike as if ready to pedal, and adjust the seat so that your leg is just slightly bent at the knee at the bottom of the pedaling motion, as you would on a regular bike. Then adjust the handlebars to an angle that feels good (you'll have to get off again to do all this). If you're planning to read or knit while you pedal, or you have an ache in your back, slant the handlebars accordingly.

2. Get back onto the bike, and get the feel of pedaling without any braking resistance at 15–20 miles (24–32 kilometers) per hour.

3. Turn up the resistance very, very slightly and pedal for 8 minutes, which is how long it takes your heart to warm up to your Fat-Burning Rate on a stationary bike. Stop and *immediately* take your pulse. If it is at your Base Fat-Burning Rate, then you should continue pedaling (at 15–20 miles per hour, no faster) for the remainder of the half-hour Session at that braking resistance. If your heart rate is not high enough, turn up the braking resistance *very slightly,* and pedal a few more minutes. Keep doing this until you reach the resistance that produces your desired heart rate. Leave the resistance there for your next Session.

Remember, you do *not* need to turn the resistance up very high to achieve the fat-burning state, especially in the first two weeks. *What seems too easy for the first 15 minutes will all of a sudden seem harder for the next 15.* If you overdo it, all you will do is poop yourself out and get discouraged. It is the *continuous nature of the effort* that gets your heart up to your Fat-Burning Rate and keeps it there. And you must give your muscles and your cardiovascular system a chance to get stronger and more efficient before they can handle more work.

Don't worry about distance, just heart rate and time. Progress at your own speed—you're not in a race! As the weeks go by, you will periodically have to do slightly more work to reach your Base (or desired) Fat-Burning Rate, because your body quickly adapts to the new demands you're putting on it. Be sure to check your pulse often—preferably at every Session in the first two weeks. If it is all of a sudden too low after you've been working at the same intensity, that's a good sign! It means your muscles and your whole body are getting more adept at burning fat. You then must encourage them to do even better by working a bit harder. The best way to do this is by turning up the braking resistance slightly, rather than increasing your speed.

Buying Information

Exercise bikes that best meet the stated requirements are the Schwinn XR-7 ($225), the Sears, Roebuck Flywheel Ergometer ($350 plus shipping), the Tunturi Home Cycle ($360) and the Tunturi Ergometer ($450). (Prices vary, so shop around.) The Schwinn and the Tunturi have been consistently praised by exercise experts and top-rated twice in *Consumer Reports* magazine. I can personally vouch for both as well, because I've used the Tunturi in many health clubs, and use a Schwinn at home.

Both models of the Tunturi are made in Finland, but are widely available throughout the United States. Both are gleaming white with chrome trim, and are sturdy and reliable. The larger of the two, the Ergometer, is truly the Mercedes of stationary biking, and allows you to scientifically measure your effort in units of work energy in addition to recording your speed and distance in kilometers. The smaller bike is just as reliable, and takes up a bit less space.

The Schwinn XR-7 is available throughout the United States only from authorized Schwinn dealers. It can be equipped with an optional reading stand (about $20—I consider it a must) and a backrest which attaches to the seat (also about $20). The bike is a handsome metallic gold with black and chrome trim.

Lazy Biking Tips

• Motivate yourself to do your Fat-Burning Session by planning it around a favorite TV show. Start pedaling when the show begins, and then you can stop when it's over. You can think of that particular program as your "Fat-Burning Show."

• Treat yourself to a special magazine for each Session, or save a juicy novel you allow yourself to read only while pedaling. You will then be eager to do your Session just so you can get to the next chapter.

• Station your bike where you will *use* it. A bike in your basement can do nothing for your fat. Don't put it in a closet, either—it's too much trouble to haul it in and out. Accept it as part of your decor.

• Turn a fan directly on yourself for summer Sessions. I

use one along with my air conditioner—and think pityingly of the joggers staggering in the heat outside.

• Treat yourself to luxurious accessories such as the reading stand and backrest (available with the Schwinn bike). An automatic pulse-rate monitor is handy too: some models are made specifically to be attached to the handlebars. I use a Pulse Tach™ Heart Computer, which is slipped periodically over one's fingertip to check heart rate and can be suspended on a string from your bike's handlebars. The Pulse Tach is available from Baystar, Dept. 19T, 110 Painters Mill Road, Owings Mills, Maryland 21117. It costs $49.95 plus $2.45 shipping charges, and may be ordered on your credit card by a phone call to 1 (800) 638-6170; Maryland residents should call 363-4304. Anything that makes fat burning more comfortable or easier for you will help you look forward to your Session.

• If your bottom isn't happy straddled that long on a bare bike seat, sit on a pillow, or make a cushion out of a towel and hold it in place with twine or a shower cap. For the ultimate in biking comfort, you can get a sheepskin seat cover (regular, not racing size), available from many biking stores. A seat cover made specially for exercise bikes is available for $12.50 postpaid from L. L. Bean, Inc., Freeport, Maine 04033—or with a credit card, 1 (207) 865-3111. Ask for the Exercycle Seat Cover.

• Give yourself a beauty treatment—such as conditioning or coloring your hair—while you pedal.

• Stock up on lots of bubble bath so you can take a luxurious relaxing soak after your Session.

2. Rebound Jogging

Another piece of legitimate and relatively inexpensive fat-burning equipment to consider is a rebounder. It's sold under many names, but basically it's a baby trampoline. The one I have is 39 inches in diameter, stands 8 inches off the floor on six legs and is very light and easy to quickly take in and out of the closet.

What do you do on a rebounder? Anything but somersaults. Just hop on and keep moving. Jogging is especially useful for fat burning, and very pleasant to do on a rebounder. Whereas indoor stationary jogging can be tedious and tends to cramp posterior thigh and calf muscles, jogging on a rebounder is very comfortable and great fun. Since it acts as a shock absorber, it does not cause the shin splits, joint pain and assorted injuries some people experience jogging on pavement. It is also not nearly as strenuous as jogging outdoors, and thus helps you get in shape much more comfortably.

A rebounder can be used anywhere there's adequate floor space—or even outdoors, if you like. No, it won't catapult you through the ceiling, because it's not quite *that* springy. But a well-made rebounder is sturdy and bouncy enough to be enjoyed by children. The only problem you may have with your rebounder is persuading your kids to let you use it once in a while.

Bouncing in Comfort

You will probably feel most comfortable wearing only shorts and a running bra, or a one-piece leotard which supports your breasts. You can wear running shoes, socks or nothing on your feet.

How to Use Your Rebounder for Successful Fat Burning

Remember, you are not limited to jogging on a rebounder. You can dance to disco music, do jumping jacks or pretend you're a Rockette. Although I mostly jog on mine, I often throw in a few other movements to keep the muscle workout balanced. Any combination of rhythmic leg movements that helps you achieve your Fat-Burning Rate is fine. (Don't get *too* carried away, however, or you can hurt yourself.)

Here's how to get started:

1. Using a watch or clock with a second hand, start jogging at a rate of 2 steps per second, or 120 steps per minute (60 per foot). Raise your feet about 8–12 inches off the rebounder as you step.

2. Jog for 3–5 minutes at that pace (which is how long it should take to reach your Base Fat-Burning Rate), then take your pulse. If it is at or above your correct rate, then jog at that pace for your first four Sessions. If your pulse is below your Base Fat-Burning Rate, you should wear 2½-pound ankle weights while you jog to increase your work effort. (You will be needing ankle weights for some of the Spot Shapers for legs in Chapter 6. See pages 122–123 for information.)

After the first two weeks, as you get more fit, you will probably need either to start wearing 2½-pound ankle weights or to graduate to heavier ones (5 pounds on each leg) to reach your correct heart rate. Check your exercise pulse periodically to see where you stand. *Special Bonus:* Wearing weights also gives all your leg muscles a terrific general firming up while you burn fat, possibly eliminating the need for other leg work.

Buying Information

Rebounders are available at many sporting-goods stores at prices from $60 to $100. Look for a sturdy steel frame and legs, heavy springs (covered with padding on top for your protection) and a tight mesh bouncing platform. Round rebounders tend to be more stable than rectangular ones.

If you can't find a rebounder locally, contact M & M Specialties, Inc., 460 East 76th Avenue, Denver, Colorado 80229, 1 (303) 287-9374 or 1 (303) 458-1078. Mine was manufactured by M & M and is very well made. The Schwinn Bicycle Company also makes a rebounder—the RB-100—which is available through Schwinn dealers. You may order a rebounder, called a Trimline Jogger Trampoline, for $69.95 plus $5.50 for shipping from The Shelburne Company, 110 Painters Mill Road, Owings Mills, Maryland 21117; call 1 (800) 638-6170 to order one on your credit card.

Lazy Bouncing Tips

• Keep your rebounder in a closet clear of junk near where you are going to use it, so you can take it in and out *easily*. If you put obstacles in the way of doing your Session, you will be less likely to do it—and your fat will stay put.

• Believe it or not, you can watch TV while bouncing up and down without getting a headache. I do it all the time.

• Disco or rock music is great to jog to. So are aerobic dance records.

• Focus a fan directly on yourself for a summer Session.

• For variety, use your rebounder outside in the fresh air.

• Make the rebounder a gift for the whole family. Every child I know loves to use mine—including me. But your kids should not try acrobatic stunts—nor should you.

3. Walking It Off

If you don't wish to purchase either a bike or a rebounder, you can use two very effective pieces of fat-burning equipment attached to your body: your feet. Even leisurely walking is a decent, if low-level, aerobic activity. In order for it to be a really effective Fat Burner, however, you must do it *briskly* and *continuously*.

Walking in Comfort

You should, of course, wear comfortable nonbinding clothes that are suitable for the weather. Do not overdress, because you will get too hot when you walk. Most imperative is a pair of comfortable shoes—preferably running shoes. Nothing can make you more miserable than blistered feet.

If you choose to walk during your lunch break at work, you probably won't want to change out of your office attire. But you can still switch from your heels into walking shoes. In Manhattan, elegant designer suits and running shoes are *de rigueur* among successful businesswomen—a fashion instituted by necessity during the last transit strike, but which has flourished since then. If you too live in a city and must walk on pavement, be sure to get running or walking shoes with extra cushioning for that purpose. A brand of running shoe I find especially good for sidewalking is Etonic.

How to Walk (Up) Right

It would seem that even lazy folks wouldn't need to be told how to walk. But if you look around you in the street, you can spot some pretty convincing arguments against bipedalism in humans. There are slouchers, shufflers and stumblers. There are those who do not look capable of standing up, much less being able to carry themselves *forward.*

You too may be guilty of "walking small," perhaps because you are overweight and self-conscious. But slumping makes you look fatter, not less noticeable. Even a very overweight person with a good posture and a cheerful, confident, proud walk looks much more attractive than a slender person who slouches and stares at her feet. Hunching over also strains weak back muscles and makes stomach muscles bulge.

To walk tall, you must first learn to stand tall. Here's how:

1. Pull shoulders back but not backward.
2. Tuck buttocks under you by rotating pelvis slightly. (This is the *opposite* of arching your back.)
3. Lift chin so you are looking straight ahead, not at your shoes.
4. Now, walk forward, taking comfortable long strides. Breathe deeply, letting your abdomen expand as you inhale—and smile.

That's how you should move—and keep moving—if you choose to use walking as your Fat Burner. (If you are plagued by an aching back and can't walk far, see Chapter 6 for special exercises.)

How to Walk for Successful Fat Burning

At the beginning of each Fat-Burning Session, walk at a moderate pace for a few minutes to warm up your heart and muscles. Then increase your speed to a level that is comfortable but feels vigorous enough to boost your heart rate sufficiently. Check your pulse after 10 minutes to see if you are at your Fat-Burning Rate. If not, increase your pace next time. If your pulse is too high, slow down. Walking up hills will, of course, greatly increase the effort and fat consumption of your Session.

If you are very badly out of shape, walking briskly or just continuously for a prolonged period may be enough to boost your pulse to your Base Fat-Burning Rate. If you are more than 25 pounds overweight, even walking slowly will be quite strenuous, because transporting your own extra weight requires extra energy. In either case, don't push too hard.

If you are under age 40 and only 10 or so pounds overweight, you may need a slight weight "handicap" to help you reach your Base Fat-Burning Rate during a 30-minute Fat-Burning Session. If you are not vain, you can wear 2½-pound ankle weights. More easily camouflaged and more comfortable is a weight belt which you can make by attaching three ankle weights together, or you can use a diver's weight belt. You need to experiment to see what weight gets your heart rate up, but 10 pounds is a good weight to start with. (See pp. 122–123 for information on buying ankle weights; a diving belt can be purchased at a sporting-goods store.) If you don't want to spend any money, just wear a backpack full of books while you walk.

As your heart and muscles grow more efficient, it will of course take more effort to boost your heart rate. This means walking faster, adding weight, or both—or simply walking for a longer period. Unless you're a race walker, walking alone won't get your heart rate into the upper end of your Fat-Burning Range (unless you're carrying a full backpack or walking around San Francisco). So at some point you may want to try a few steps (just a few!) of jogging interspersed with brisk walking. But you don't ever have to become an official jogger. Just keep those feet moving continuously *somehow*. And if you don't want to bother with weights, you can simply get out there and walk for the pleasure of it. A comfortable 3-mile-an-hour pace will get most unconditioned people's heart rates up to 50–60 percent of maximum—still enough to give you all the fat-burning benefits. If you are sure to cover 3 miles, you will burn approximately 300 calories per Session.

Lazy Walking Tips

• Buy a pedometer to check your mileage. Look for one that can be adjusted for your stride length. It's fun to see the miles pile up. In six weeks, you'll be surprised to see how far you've come—and gone.

• Use your car odometer to trace courses exactly 1½ miles away from your home in a couple of different directions.

Note the tree or house that marks the distance. You can then choose the course that suits your fancy each day—and you can be sure you have completed 3 miles simply by returning home again. Take a different route each day, so you won't get bored.

• Become an explorer. Hike to unfamiliar places in your neighborhood.

• A good way to get your Fat-Burning Session in during a busy day is to walk to or from work, if at all possible. Leave a pair of walking shoes in your office so you can walk home when the weather's nice.

• If you have a lunch hour, walk for half of it, preferably with a co-worker who also wants to burn fat. Then have lunch. Or have a light lunch first, and walk for "dessert."

• Take a child on your walk. Children from the age of 3 on can, with a bit of encouragement, keep up with an adult and walk 5 miles or more with no problem. Being used to riding everywhere, your child may whine at first. If you must coax your tot to accompany you on your walk, pack an occasional surprise in a backpack. Tell the child that when you have reached the "halfway point" in your walk he or she will get the surprise. There is nothing wrong with bribes if they pave the road to good health!

• If you have more than one young child, walk with a different one each day. That way, the child will feel she or he has a special private time with you. By getting your kids to walk, you are setting a precedent for physical activity in their lives that will *forever* prevent them from being fat.

• If you have a baby or toddler, push her or him in a stroller. That may be all you need to get your heart rate up and to calm your cranky offspring.

• Buy a Sony Walkman–type cassette player with headphones and a few of your favorite music tapes to walk to.

• If you need to carry weight to get your heart rate up, use a backpack and fill it with a thermos of water or juice, some fruit and a book. That way, when you reach your destination you can rest and have refreshment at hand. This is especially helpful if you are going on a country walk.

• Instead of having a fattening coffee-and-Danish break with a friend, have a fat-burning break. (You can easily gossip while you walk—remember, you're doing "conversational" exercise!) Or encourage a group of neighborhood friends to join you.

• Pack a pair of comfortable shoes and walk everywhere on your vacation. It's the best way to see the sights, and to burn off all those delicious meals.

• Your dog would love to go for a walk, and doubtless can use the exercise as much as you can. Or buy a dog so you have a good reason to walk.

GENERAL GUIDELINES: YOUR FAT-BURNING "BREAKTHROUGH"

After perhaps the sixth Fat-Burning Session, you may start to feel as if you're doing nothing: a constant amount of resistance or weight or speed will simply be too easy. That's the time to be sure to check your pulse while you're doing your Session, to make sure you're at least at your Base Fat-Burning Rate. If not, increase your work load slightly until you get it back up there.

A body that has been underutilized for many years *initially* responds to training by getting into better condition quite quickly. That's why you'll notice the characteristic "break-through" somewhere in the second week of your Sessions. At that point, you'll increase your work load a bit (with braking resistance or weights) so you can progress further. You will improve a bit more, and then work a little more.

Always give yourself just enough of an "overload" to keep your muscles and all fat-burning systems sufficiently stimulated. You can, of course, do this just by making sure your Sessions are always done at or above your Base Fat-Burning Rate. But your body thrives on stimulation, so it's a good idea to do a more challenging Fat-Burning Session perhaps once a week, during which you push your heart rate up fairly high within your Fat-Burning Range. You can simply do a longer Session—say, 45 minutes to an hour. Or you can do five instead of four Fat-Burning Sessions at your Base Fat-Burning Rate.

So if, after three weeks or so, you feel you can do more, by all means *do* it. I know you don't believe it now, but if you get through the first two weeks, you will actually get *hooked* on fat burning: on some days, you simply won't feel satisfied with 30 minutes. There are, in fact, powerful substances that begin to be manufactured in large quantities by the body after 45 minutes of fat burning which have a dramatic calming effect on the emotions. These substances, the endorphins and enkephalins, are the body's own natural tranquilizers and painkillers—and they are 10 times as powerful as morphine! So the making of your better body can be a *very* pleasurable addiction.

Whether or not you stick to the basic four-day 30-minute Session schedule, you can always rely on feedback from your body as your guide to successful fat burning. Remember, good Sessions should never leave you gasping for breath or feeling faint. But they will soon leave you much leaner!

5 / The Better Body Diet

Besides what diets do to your body, there's another compelling reason they don't work: they make you hungry. Eating is one of life's great sensual pleasures. Not eating (or eating painfully small amounts of unappetizing foods) is cruel and unusual punishment. After two days on nothing but hard-boiled eggs and dry toast, one is invariably transformed into a ravenous beast capable of devouring an entire cheesecake in one gulp.

Besides that, being a cook, food writer and dedicated eater who has had the privilege of serving as an unofficial Assistant Palate to one of the nation's leading restaurant critics (I shall always treasure memories of the Night of the Six Chocolate Desserts), I am hardly one to urge you to give up lasagne or cut rations to a few miserable crumbs.

The purpose of this chapter, therefore, is obviously not to introduce you to yet another creative way to starve yourself. Nor are you going to be put on a joyless regimen of such "health" foods as soybeans and yeast—because *all* good food is by definition health food. And unless your idea of breakfast is a couple of Twinkies washed down with a quart of Coke, you don't even have to eliminate all your favorite foods. In fact, you'll be encouraged to eat things you never thought you could eat while *still* losing weight.

Of course, after the haranguing about the horrors of dieting you've already received, it may seem hypocritical of me to *present* you with a diet. But that information pertains to dieting *while remaining sedentary*—something you won't be doing on the Plan.

When you are on a moderately reduced-calorie, nutritious and balanced diet such as the Better Body Diet, along with doing your Fat-Burning Sessions, the internal situation changes completely. Your basal metabolic rate remains normal. Instead of losing your precious, fat-hungry muscle tissue, you preserve it and even build more. Calories get continuously burned around the clock. Best of all, your fat drops off with amazing speed. Fat-burning activity and sensible dieting is the most effective combination there is for building a better body.

The basic Better Body Diet provides you with approximately 1200 calories per day. That's the magic minimum that can provide all the nutrients the average adult female *must* have to stay healthy and energetic while maximizing fat loss and also leaving room for the soul-satisfying treats and indulgences that keep you happy.

Keeping you happy—and full—is the secret of this diet's success. You know how often in the past you abandoned a diet when your stomach began to growl and you felt deprived of too many pleasures. So you won't be making any tasteless "diet" recipes. You can have some fat and sugar. You are actually *encouraged* to eat snacks, and can even choose an occasional treat—such as chocolates or champagne—from a special "Splurge List." You can afford such extravagances because your diet is composed *primarily* of foods that had to meet some special nutritional requirements in order to be included. Filling your daily menu with such foods is the key not only to losing weight on the Plan, but also to staying slim permanently.

MAKING EVERY CALORIE COUNT

The calories you need to keep you going each day can't be any old calories you find lying around the kitchen. They must be calories of the key nutrients protein, carbohydrate and fat, which must also bring in vitamins and minerals along with them. If you consume your calories in the form of foods that have little to offer *but* empty concentrated calories, or too many calories of one nutrient at the expense of other nutrients, you are cheating your body of the fuel, building material and other substances that it needs to operate in top form. You will be tired and irritable—along with staying fat.

Say, for example, you have two doughnuts and black coffee for breakfast, and a cheeseburger and fries for lunch. In order not to gain weight—you've already consumed a lot of calories—you skimp on dinner. You may not gain weight, but you have not filled most of your nutritional requirements. If you go ahead and have a big dinner—steak, a vegetable, dessert—you may have added a few more nutrients, but you have gone over your maintenance calorie quota. In either case, you have dined poorly.

In order to be well nourished without getting fat, you must construct your daily menu of foods that give you plenty of nutrition for relatively few calories. While you are maintaining your weight, your first choice should always be such foods. Then, as long as you have filled your nutritional requirements and still have room within your weight-maintenance calorie quota, you can also enjoy that luscious piece of chocolate cake.

But on a weight-reduction diet, you obviously don't have

as many calories to play with. It is therefore absolutely critical that you "spend" all your caloric dollars wisely. Although
you are trimming calories a bit, your body's minimum requirements for protein, carbohydrates, fat, vitamins and minerals don't change. So the foods you must reach for almost ex-
clusively on a reduced-calorie regimen are those which have
high *nutrient density*.

Foods with the highest nutrient density are those which
offer the most impressive list of nutrients—protein, carbohydrates, vitamins and minerals—for the fewest calories. They
are also foods which offer the least natural or added fat, because fat invariably means calories. And they are foods that
have little or no added sugar.

Now here comes the great news: some of the least fattening, most filling, best nutrient "bargains" around are the very
foods you've always loved but thought were the most fattening: carbohydrates!

GETTING SLIM ON STARCH

Yes, all the wonderful starchy foods you were brainwashed
into feeling guilty about eating by many popular fad diets of
the last decade are the very foods that can get you and keep
you skinny. Such foods as potatoes, rice, corn, beans, bread,
cereals and even spaghetti are a very important part of your
Better Body Diet. In fact, you're *required* to eat at least five
servings a day of any kind of starchy food you want!

How can this be true? First of all, the main ingredient in
these foods, starch, is the ideal energy food for your body.
Starch is a "complex" carbohydrate—a chain of simple
sugars which breaks down to provide a rich and steady source
of the glucose your body needs to run on every day. An ample
supply of carbohydrates ensures that protein will be spared

from energy production and instead be used properly to build new lean tissues. A diet high in carbohydrate foods also alters brain chemistry, increasing the quantity of serotonin, a neurotransmitter that elevates mood, making you feel better. What's more, carbohydrates must be present to help fat break down all the way, acting as the "match" that sets fat on fire. The best and healthiest way for you to lose fat happily *and* fast, then, is to eat plenty of spaghetti!

While you can save all the starch servings on your diet for that occasional pasta feast, you should usually try to eat a variety of starchy foods each day, including at least one starchy vegetable such as peas, potatoes or corn, plus grain products. You may eat any kind of bread or unsweetened cereal you want for energy. (As you'll note on your food lists, you can even have an occasional doughnut, a piece of cake or some cookies.) But you should try to have at least three servings of whole-wheat or other whole-grain bread and/or cereal products per day, as they supply a host of B vitamins and minerals missing from refined-white-flour products. It is the B vitamins that are in charge of energy production in your cells. So if you want fat to burn off at top speed, you should fill up on bran muffins, whole-wheat bread or whole-wheat pasta, and corn tortillas.

The other complex-carbohydrate foods which make up a major part of the Better Body Diet are vegetables and fruit. Crunchy, colorful vegetables, along with the starchy foods, are the reasons you won't ever go hungry on your diet, because you can eat many of them in virtually unlimited quantities. You will also be eating three servings of fruit per day. Both vegetables and fruits supply vital vitamins and minerals, and energy in the form of sugar. Fruit especially is the natural nutrient-dense way to satisfy your sweet tooth.

Along with their abundance of nutrients, all the above foods contain an additional substance that can't be digested but is *critical* to fat loss, and which is very likely lacking in your current diet: fiber.

The Fat Sponges

You may have heard that fiber is good for you because it acts as a sort of internal "housekeeper," helping to keep things moving through your intestinal tract. But it can also help you lose fat faster. Since fiber absorbs water and becomes bulky, foods containing fiber make you feel full for relatively fewer calories than fiberless foods that are concentrated forms of calories, such as fat, sugar and refined-flour products. That is why a bran muffin is more stomach-filling (as well as more nutritious) than a plain cake doughnut, even if both contain the same number of calories. For this reason alone, you should always have raw vegetables, whole-wheat or bran crackers or popcorn to nibble on while you are on the diet.

Beyond that, however, fiber has a unique talent for actually *preventing* some calories you consume from being absorbed. Recent studies have shown that fruits, vegetables and grains especially high in fiber act like tiny "Fat Sponges," absorbing up to 150 calories' worth of food each day and eliminating them from your body. That's 150 calories that didn't have a chance to be digested and turned into fat—a total of a third of a pound a week that otherwise would have ended up in fat cells!

The upshot is that a high-fiber diet is actually less fattening than the low-fiber diet you're eating now, *even if it contains the same number of calories.* Increasing the Fat Sponge content of your diet doesn't mean you can eat a quarter-pound of butter every day and expect it to slip unheralded by your hips. What it does mean is that you will "waste" more calories on a diet containing lots of fiber than on one that is low in fiber.

Fresh raw whole fruits and vegetables are the best sources of "Fat Sponge" fiber, as are whole-grain bread or cereal products. While you shouldn't feel compelled to eat orange peels or seeds, be sure to eat the palatable skins of fruits and vegetables, because that's where most of the fiber as well as the vitamins and minerals are found. You'll find a symbol indicating especially effective Fat Sponge foods on the food lists for your diet.

PROTEIN

Protein is the structural material out of which most of you is made, including muscles, skin, internal organs, bones, hair and nails. To maintain these tissues, as well as create blood and enzymes, you must have a small amount of protein—about 1½ ounces for the average woman—from all food sources in your diet every day.

If some protein is good, more must be better, right? No. Overdosing on protein, which many people do these days, is very bad for you. It puts a strain on your liver and kidneys, and weakens your bones by robbing them of calcium. And if too much of that protein is consumed (as it often is) in the form of beef or whole-milk dairy products, a lot of unhealthful saturated fat comes along with it.

Red meat is an excellent source of protein as well as an important source of the iron and zinc needed by many women. On the Better Body Diet, you may have up to 6 ounces of meat, fish or chicken each day. But you should know that these foods aren't the only sources of protein available to you: starchy and other vegetables, grains, beans, low- or nonfat dairy products and egg whites also contain protein along with little or no fat, which is why vegetarians can stay perfectly healthy and slim. You get more than enough protein on your diet from the combination of the animal and vegetable foods you'll be eating without going overboard on fattening forms of meat products. Relying more often on starchy vegetables, grains, beans and low-fat dairy products for protein is a very good way to automatically cut down on fat and calories, and is a habit you should get into that can help you stay svelte forever, as well as lessening your risk of cardiovascular diseases and cancer.

SUGAR

A sweet tooth is very likely inborn—which makes sense, because the sweetest things in nature, fruits, are good for you.

Contrary to faddish health notions, sugar is not poison. The carbohydrates found in fruits and vegetables are mostly simple sugars similar to table sugar. But processed foods, candies, baked goods, and your morning coffee often provide more sugar and refined starch unaccompanied by other nutrients than your body was designed to handle at once, which can be quite fattening. A dose of pure sugar such as you get in a soft drink enters your bloodstream very rapidly. This unaccustomed sugar flood stimulates a rush of insulin from your pancreas, which has the job of letting sugar into your body cells to be used for energy. Once the cells have taken in all the sugar they can use (which isn't much if you're sedentary), the rest is made into fat, much of which is sent to fat cells for storage; some may hang around and coat the insides of your arteries. (This doesn't happen as easily with starchy complex carbohydrate foods that contain fiber; they are broken down more slowly and can be gradually burned for energy before being made into fat. When this happens, your *normal* blood sugar also gets caught in the rush and may drop way down for hours, making you feel tired. You also get abnormally hungry, especially for sweet foods (or anything you can get your hands on), even if your stomach is full. This is a depressingly common merry-go-round syndrome of the binging sweets eater, and the bane of the sufferer from hypoglycemia, or chronic low blood sugar.

You may be impatiently muttering that you use artificial sweeteners in your coffee and always drink diet soda. Whether you continue to do so is up to you. Unfortunately, there is no evidence that people who regularly use artificial sweeteners or swig Tab are any slimmer than those who don't. (After all, are *you* as slim as you ought to be right now?) The excuse that you'd be even *fatter* if you used sugar doesn't wash either. How many times have you ordered pecan pie à la mode for dessert, only to put Sweet 'n Low in your coffee?

By using saccharin, you are also introducing yet another possibly cancer-causing chemical into your body, which I prefer not to do. (So far, no one has proved that a little sucrose once in a while causes anything worse than cavities and plump thighs in well-nourished, nondiabetic, nonhypoglycemic, otherwise healthy people.) If you have a really *insatiable* sweet tooth, you may wish to switch to aspartame, which is a sweetener made of two amino acids found naturally in berries and other plants. It is now being offered in a product called Equal™ from the G. D. Searle drug company. Equal™ contains a small amount of lactose, or milk sugar, along with aspartame, but it amounts to only about 2 calories per teaspoon. I have tasted it, and it is far superior to saccharin in that it tastes like sugar and leaves no aftertaste. It will soon be found in diet soft drinks. One drawback is that you cannot cook with it, because it is destroyed by heat.

Whatever you decide, remember that the overuse of artificial sweeteners will still perpetuate exaggerated craving for sweetness, which invariably encourages periodic binges on

The Real Thing. It is best by far to learn to consume sugar rationally.

So you can have a little sugar in your life and on your diet and not feel guilty. After the first week, you may choose to add up to two teaspoons of sugar, syrup or honey to your daily menu (as long as it fits in your calorie quota for the day and is not substituted for real food). And you get to choose an occasional sweet treat from the Splurge List, too. But always remember to reach for fruit first when you want something sweet, both on your diet and from now on. Save sugar for special occasions rather than mindlessly sprinkling it everywhere.

FAT

As you well know, an excess of calories beyond what your body can use each day of any calorie-containing nutrient—protein, carbohydrate or fat—will be converted into body fat. Once body fat is formed out of any nutrient, it cannot be changed back into that nutrient—meaning that you *must* have sufficient protein and carbohydrates in your daily diet no matter how overfat you are. And virtually the only use of extra body fat is for fuel.

But right now, you are no doubt getting many hundreds of extra fat calories in your daily diet, from the visible sources you add to food yourself, such as butter, oil and mayonnaise; from the fat naturally found in foods or added to processed foods; and from beef, as well as from candy, pastries and junky snack and fast foods. While protein and carbohydrates (including plain sugar) contain only 4 calories per gram, fat supplies a whopping 9 *calories per gram.* So fat is truly the most fattening thing you can eat.

Like sugar, fat tastes good. And you do need some fat in your diet each day, to supply one important fatty acid that you can't make in your body and to serve as a medium through which certain fat-soluble vitamins can be used by your body. But the amount of daily dietary fat needed by the average woman for these essential functions is *very small*— only about 100–200 calories' worth. If you never consciously added fat to your food and simply ate a balanced diet, you would still be getting all you needed, because so many foods contain some fat in their natural state—including the leanest meats.

Beyond your minimal fat requirement, extra fat has no other purpose and instantly heads straight for your fat cells. The fat you consume can, of course, be burned for energy— but the point is to get rid of your *body* fat first.

It is therefore essential for you to learn to control your fat intake both while you're trying to lose weight and to stay slim. This means keeping track of visible fat sources as well as foods that have a hidden high fat content. The Fat Source list in the Diet section of this chapter helps you learn how to spot specific amounts of fat on sight so you will always know approximately how much fat you're getting even while dining out.

For the first week of your diet, you will not be using any added fat in your food. This will dramatically speed your fat loss. If you continue to eat "fat-free" for the entire six weeks, you will continue to lose fat at a very fast rate. After week one, you have the option of adding up to 100 calories, or approximately 1 tablespoon, of butter, margarine, oil or mayonnaise (or an equivalent high-fat food source), to your menu occasionally or daily for the remainder of your diet. But remember—the less fat you use, the more you'll lose.

VITAMINS AND MINERALS: WHAT YOU
SHOULDN'T BE MISSING

By eating the amount of whole-grain products suggested on your diet plus meat and vegetables, you will get B vitamins along with important trace minerals. You will be able to fill your requirements for vitamins A and C by eating at least one citrus and/or yellow-fleshed fruit (cantaloupe, peaches, apricots) per day and at least one dark green vegetable (spinach, kale, broccoli) or one yellow vegetable (carrots, yams, winter squash) per day. (White potatoes, by the way, are also a good source of vitamin C.) Fat-soluble vitamins E and K are available in many of the above foods. Vitamin D, also fat-soluble, is obtained through exposure of fair skin to sunlight or consumption of small amounts of low-fat dairy products.

Calcium deficiency has emerged as a major nutritional problem in women. Whether you are dieting or not, you must get enough calcium to maintain a strong skeleton. Without it, you are setting the stage for osteoporosis, the disease characterized by thinning and brittleness of bones that is beginning to plague more and more women. Osteoporosis can be recognized by the dowager's hump of advanced age, but most often it is invisible—until a fall happens and the bones snap like matchsticks. It was until recently thought to be caused almost entirely by an estrogen deficiency that occurs at menopause. But inadequate calcium intake throughout life and a lack of bone-stressing exercise have emerged as by far the most important causes. (And studies have shown that loss of spinal bone tissue doesn't happen suddenly in middle age, but begins as early as *age 20!*)

Your Fat-Burning Sessions provide the proper stimulation your bones need to stay strong. But an occasional container of yogurt is not enough to meet your requirement for calcium. Experts currently recommend that daily calcium intake should be 1000 milligrams per day for women under 35, and 1500 milligrams for women 35 and over. The best sources of calcium are dairy products such as milk or yogurt (240 milligrams per cup) and cheese (200 milligrams per ounce; skim or low-fat is preferred, since fat binds with calcium and prevents its absorption by the body, and you don't need the fat calories); salmon and sardines with bones (60 and 100 milligrams per ounce respectively); broccoli (150 milligrams per large stalk) and dark leafy greens (200 milligrams per cup cooked or tightly packed raw). If you are under 35, you will be able to get sufficient calcium on the diet from your two servings of skim or low-fat milk and by regularly including enough of the other foods mentioned—especially a few cups of those low-cal, nutrient-dense greens—in your daily menu. You can also easily boost calcium intake by adding nonfat dry milk powder to baked goods or skim-milkshakes. If you are 35 or over, can't tolerate dairy products or can't conceive of eating enough of the other foods listed to compensate, experts recommend that you take calcium carbonate (not calcium gluconate or calcium lactate) supplements, such as Os Cal 500 by Marion Laboratories. (Do *not*, however, overdose on calcium supplements, as this may cause kidney stones or other problems. Take only as much as you need to fill your age-related requirement.) If you don't regularly consume dairy products, you should also be sure to take a multivitamin containing vitamin D.

Iron carries oxygen to your cells to help them use energy, so not having enough will indeed make you feel pooped. An iron deficiency is most common in women of menstruating age, who require 18 milligrams a day. On your diet, you should be getting enough if you have regular twice-weekly servings of red meat and/or liver, as well as beans, plenty of dark green leafy vegetables, whole-grain products, and dried fruit. If you have especially heavy periods, feel free to take a 30-milligram iron supplement (no more), at least during menstruation.

The vitamin folacin (folic acid) and the mineral zinc may also be lacking in your diet. Folacin is found in liver and dark leafy greens, and zinc is found in meat, liver, eggs, poultry and shellfish.

Should you take a daily multivitamin-and-mineral supplement? Nutritionists and physicians today are becoming increasingly concerned that deficiencies other than those already mentioned occur even if one is consuming a "balanced" diet, owing to nutrient-depleting processing and shipping of food, pollution, illness and a history of poor eating habits, among other environmental and personal factors. Some experts claim that the RDAs are grossly inadequate for most people. Vitamins and minerals are also being recognized as potent disease-fighting agents; vitamin A (specifically in its nontoxic plant-derived form, beta-carotene), vitamin C and the minerals selenium and zinc are currently being studied in an effort to ascertain their role in preventing and even curing heart disease and cancer. So taking at least a daily high-potency multivitamin-mineral supplement definitely can't hurt you, and is strongly recommended while you're dieting. (Do not take additional vitamin A or D above the amount found in your supplement, however, as they can be toxic.) But you should not rely solely on pills to give you what you need. Nor do they give you an excuse to eat only junk food! Vitamins and minerals work in concert; leave out the violins and your metabolic symphony won't play. Only a rich variety of fresh, minimally doctored foods can give you a spectrum of vitamins and minerals and the protein, carbohydrates, fatty acids and fiber you need for optimum health.

SALT

Salt doesn't actually make you fat, because it has no calories. But eating too much salt can mess up your body's natural water balance. In its attempt to dilute the unnaturally high concentration of salt in your tissues, your body holds on to extra water, which in turn makes you bloated. Since water is very heavy and takes up room, you look and feel fat and, of course, weigh more. This can be especially bothersome around your period, because the female hormones active at that time also attract water like magnets.

Most people eat 20 times the salt they need. Try to use salt sparingly. Don't automatically salt your food before you taste it. Use spices and herbs instead. And read labels—anything containing sodium means salt. You might use the next few weeks to gradually wean yourself from the craving for too much salt, as you will be doing with sugar and fat. (If you watch salt and sugar intake and still have a problem with water retention, be sure to see your doctor.)

WATER

Your entire body is at least 50 percent water; your muscles, even more. Without enough water, your skin will look lousy and you will be weak and feel tired. You also need water to keep your intestinal pipes clean. Oddly, getting enough water will also help prevent you from retaining it. When your body is dehydrated, it desperately tries to hang on to its precious remaining water supply, and may hoard it in unattractive places, such as your ankles. So you should drink a lot of it. Instead of diet sodas (which may contain bloat-promoting sodium saccharin), drink plain water with a slice of lemon, fruit juice, fruit syrup mixed with soda water—or just plain water.

ALCOHOL

Alcohol can be considered a carbohydrate, because once drunk, it behaves like an infusion of sugar, entering the bloodstream very quickly and expecting to be used as energy. This is seldom the case, since the drinker doesn't usually feel like a brisk walk at that point, so the unused calories usually head for fat cells.

Having a drink, of course, is one of life's pleasures. The Splurge List on your diet provides for an occasional cocktail or glass of wine—if you can stop at just one. Unfortunately, alcohol is a potent appetite stimulant and can therefore make you eat too much of all the wrong things. If it doesn't affect you like that, you can, if you wish, have one drink made with 1½ ounces of Scotch, vodka, gin, etc., or one 4-ounce glass of red or white wine in place of 1 tablespoon, or 100 calories, of fat any night, or every night. But alcohol must *never, never* take the place of nutritious foods! Do feel free to cook with wine or liquor, however, because the calories evaporate in the heat. And fresh fruit marinated in a dash of liqueur makes an elegant low-calorie dessert.

SNACKS CAN MAKE YOU SLIM

Every time you eat anything, your digestive machinery must be turned on, which uses energy. So the more often you eat, the more calories you use up. That means snacking isn't the downfall of the dieter—it's the best possible way to keep your fat fires burning! On your diet, therefore, you should try to spread your calories out so you can eat at least two snacks in addition to three meals. Use the suggested Snack List, or make up your own. Just make sure that the total calories you eat each day add up to 1200. Always.

The Better Body Diet: Getting Started

The basic 1200-calorie diet gives you all the nutrients and fiber you need to build your better body by having you construct your daily menu of the following portions of various foods:

5 servings of starches
6 servings of protein sources
2 or more servings of vegetables
3 servings of fruit
2 servings of dairy products
3 servings of fat (totaling 1 tablespoon or 100 calories)
2 servings of sugar (2 teaspoons)

You may put these foods together in any way you want, including in your favorite recipes, as long as you have an idea of how much of each food serving you're getting in each portion.

For the first week, you may wish to use the 1000-Calorie Fat Loss Booster Diet. It is the same as the basic diet except that it does not include the servings of added fat or sugar as noted above. It will get your fat loss off to a dramatic and speedy start.

Fat and sugar are, of course, always optional. If you don't wish to use one or the other or both throughout your diet (or on any particular day), you have the option of adding to your menu an extra serving of starch, an extra serving of a low-fat dairy product or another serving or two of fruit, or any combination of the above that adds the 200 calories needed to total 1200 calories. This gives you a great deal of flexibility in planning your menu. And you'll find that if you do leave added fat out of your menu more often than not, you will lose weight faster.

You can expect to lose anywhere from 3 to 6 pounds during Week One of the Plan. This is due in part to the usual temporary water loss that happens on any diet. But part of that is also the solid fat weight you'll be losing from day one, thanks to your Fat-Burning Sessions—which, in turn, also make your diet work properly. From then on, you can expect to lose 1–2 pounds per week of pure fat. But you *must* be patient with yourself. Dramatic, quick weight loss in the past may have spoiled you—but as we all know, that loss did not last.

DIETING THE LAZY WAY

For maximum convenience, I have organized the Better Body Diet into seven general Food Categories: Starches, Protein Sources, Vegetables, Fruits, Dairy Products, Fat Sources and Sugars. Each category is composed of specific portions of food that all contain approximately the same number of calories. This eliminates the tedious weighing and measuring that may have bogged you down during so many diets past. In the beginning it may help you to learn what, say, 3 ounces of meat or a cup of cooked pasta looks like on your plate. But once you do so, and familiarize yourself with what constitutes a serving of all similar foods in a category, you don't have to count a single calorie—you just keep track of servings. (No one—not even a nutritionist—can accurately count calories anyway.) But do always watch fat intake; an extra slice of bread can't slow fat loss nearly as much as an extra blob of mayo!

Each category also features special symbols which guide you toward foods that you need to choose regularly to help fill your all-important daily requirements for critical vitamins and minerals. The best high-fiber, Fat Sponge foods are also indicated.

Following the food lists, you'll find suggested meal plans. They aren't rigid menus you must stick to. Rather, they show you what common foods and dishes can readily be included in your diet. Since so many people eat at least one meal out these days, I've also included guidelines for restaurant and bag-lunch dining. At the end of the chapter, you'll find tips on preparing food that prove you can spare the fat (and sugar) without spoiling the flavor. Making them part of your permanent cooking repertoire will assure you of always being able to eat well while remaining slim.

The ultimate pleasant surprise you probably haven't encountered on a diet before is the special Splurge List. It is blatantly designed to keep you motivated, and is composed of items with little or no redeeming nutritional value, one of which you are to consume, out of sheer perversity, every three days. You may feel free to enjoy any one of the 100-calorie items listed, be it champagne, caviar, chocolates or the disgustingly gloppy treat of your choice. (Yes, you can even have—God forbid—a Twinkie, if you so desire, as long as you pledge to enjoy it immensely and feel suitably wicked. Licking fingers is mandatory.)

So there's no need to go hungry or get bored on the Better Body Diet. Between all the starches and snacks and splurges, in fact, you'll hardly know you're on a diet at all!

FOOD CATEGORY 1: STARCHES

Servings per day: 5 including 3 servings of whole-wheat or other whole-grain products, and 1 serving of a starchy vegetable
Calories per serving: about 70

> **KEY**
> ☻ —Fat Sponge
> ●━● —Iron Source
> ⋈ —Calcium Source

BREADS

White, ☻ ●━● whole-wheat, raisin	1 slice
Bread crumbs, dry	3 tbs.
Breadsticks	3
Bread stuffing	¼ cup
Biscuit, dinner roll	1 small
Bun, hamburger, hot dog	½
Cake, angel food, sponge	1 thin slice
⋈ Corn bread	1 small cube
English muffin, bagel, ☻ whole-wheat, white	½
Matzoh, ☻ whole-wheat, white	¾
Muffin, ●━● ☻ bran, ⋈ corn	1 small
Pancake, waffle, ☻ ●━● whole-wheat, white	1
Pita, ☻ ●━● whole-wheat, white	1 small
Tortilla, ☻ corn, flour	1 small

CEREALS

●━● ☻ Cereal, whole-grain, oatmeal, cooked	½ cup
●━● ☻ Cereal, ready-to-eat, whole-grain, unsweetened	¾ cup

●━● ⊕	Bran	5 tbs.
●━● ⊕	Bran flakes	½ cup
	Dry, puffed	1½ cups
	Cornmeal, dry	2 tbs.
	Cornstarch	2 tbs.
	Flour, white, ⊕ whole-wheat	2½ tbs.
●━● ⊕	Wheat germ	2 tbs.

CRACKERS

Plain, butter-type	5
Graham	2 squares
Melba toast	5
Rye wafers	3
Saltines	6
Vanilla wafers	5
⊕ Whole-wheat crackers	8 small

STARCHY VEGETABLES

⊕ Corn	½ cup
⊕ Corn on the cob	1 small ear
⊕ Lima beans	½ cup
Parsnips	¾ cup
⊕ Peas, green, fresh, canned or frozen	½ cup
⊕ Potato, white, with skin	1 small
Potato, mashed	½ cup
⊕ Winter squash, acorn, butternut	½ cup
⊕ Yam or sweet potato	¼ cup

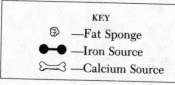

```
                    KEY
        ⊕    —Fat Sponge
       ●━●   —Iron Source
       ⊂⊃    —Calcium Source
```

PASTA

Spaghetti, macaroni, all
shapes & sizes, white,
●━● ⊕ whole-wheat, vegetable, cooked   ½ cup
Egg noodles, cooked   ½ cup

DRIED BEANS, PEAS, LENTILS

●━● ⊕ Beans, peas, lentils, dried,
     cooked   ½ cup
●━● ⊕ Baked beans, no pork   ¼ cup
●━● ⊕ Pea soup   ½ cup

WHOLE GRAINS

●━● ⊕ Barley   ½ cup
●━● ⊕ Bulgar (cracked wheat)   ½ cup
●━● ⊕ Kasha (buckwheat), Rice,
     ●━● ⊕ brown,   ½ cup
●━● ⊕ All other grains   ½ cup

STARCHY TREATS
(for occasional consumption)

⊕ Corn chips (no more than one
     serving per day)   1-oz. bag
⊕ Popcorn, air-popped   3 cups
French fries (no more than 2
servings per day; use no other
fat if more than 1 serving per
day consumed)   8 medium

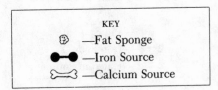

KEY	
⊕	—Fat Sponge
●━●	—Iron Source
⊂⊐	—Calcium Source

Potato chips (no more than 2 servings per day)	15
Pretzels, thin sticks	25
⊕ Seeds—squash, pumpkin, sunflower, with or without shells	1 small handful

FOOD CATEGORY 2: PROTEIN SOURCES

Servings per day: 6
Calories per serving: about 55

Colds cuts, sliced thin: *salami, *bologna, *liverwurst, ●━━● roast beef, ham, chicken, turkey	1 slice
●━━● ⊕ Dried beans, lentils, peas, cooked	½ cup
Egg	1
Fish, shellfish: fresh or frozen cod, flounder, haddock, etc.	1 oz.
⊂⟩ Salmon, tuna, crab, water pack	¼ cup
Tuna in oil, well drained	¼ cup
Lobster	1 tail
⊂⟩ Oysters, shrimps, clams, scallops	5

*This is high in fat and calories. Have no more than 1 serving per week.

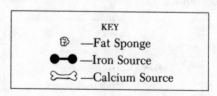

```
                    KEY
        ⊕   —Fat Sponge
        ●━━●—Iron Source
        ⊂⟩ —Calcium Source
```

≈⊃ Sardines (packed in water,
mustard, tomato sauce or oil,
well-rinsed)　　　　　　3 medium
Meat and poultry:
●—● beef, veal, ●—● lamb,
　●—● pork, ●—● liver,
chicken, turkey, etc., lean and
trimmed of all fat and/or skin　　1 oz.
*Frankfurter　　　　　　　1
*Sausage, small　　　　　　1
Peanut butter　　　　　　　2 tsp.

FOOD CATEGORY 3: VEGETABLES

Servings per day: 2 or more, including at least one dark green leafy,
　　　　dark green and/or yellow-orange vegetable
Calories per ½-cup serving: 25

Asparagus	≈⊃ ●—● Dark, leafy greens:
Bean sprouts	beet
Beets	chard
≈⊃ ●—● ⊕ Broccoli	collard
⊕ Brussels sprouts	dandelion
⊕ Cabbage	kale
⊕ Carrots	mustard
Cauliflower	spinach
Eggplant	turnip
⊕ Green pepper	Mushrooms

*This is high in fat and calories. Have no more than 1 serving per week.

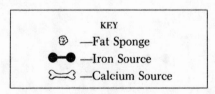

KEY
⊕　—Fat Sponge
●—●　—Iron Source
≈⊃　—Calcium Source

Okra
Rhubarb
Rutabaga (yellow
   turnips)
Sauerkraut
String beans,
   green or yellow

Summer squash
Tomatoes
Tomato juice
Tomato sauce
Turnips
Vegetable juice
Zucchini

UNLIMITED VEGETABLES

Celery, raw
Chicory
Chinese cabbage
Cucumbers
Endive

Escarole
Lettuce
Onions
Radishes
Watercress

FOOD CATEGORY 4: FRUITS

Servings per day:	3, including at least 1 citrus and/or orange/ yellow-fleshed fruit
Calories per serving:	40

Apple   1 small
Applesauce (unsweetened)   ½ cup
Apricots, fresh   2 medium
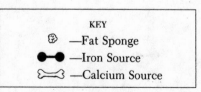 Apricots, dried   4 halves
Banana   ½

KEY
🕸 —Fat Sponge
●—● —Iron Source
〰 —Calcium Source

✪ Berries:

Blackberries	½ cup
Blueberries	½ cup
Raspberries	⅔ cup
Strawberries	¾ cup
Cherries	10 large
✪ Cranberries	1 cup
✪ Dates	2
●━● ✪ Figs, dried	1
Figs, fresh	1
Grapfruit	½
Grapes	12
Kiwi fruit	2
Mango	½
Melon:	
Cantaloupe	¼
Honeydew	⅛
Watermelon	1 cup
Nectarine	1 small
Orange	1 small
Papaya	1 small
✪ Peach	1
✪ Pear	1
Persimmon	1
Pineapple	½ cup, 1 ring
Plums	2
●━● ✪ Prunes	2
●━● ✪ Raisins	2 tbs.
Tangerine	1

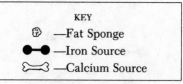

KEY

✪ —Fat Sponge

●━● —Iron Source

〔⟋〕 —Calcium Source

FRUIT JUICES

Apple	⅓ cup
Cider	⅓ cup
Cranberry	½ cup
Grapefruit	½ cup
Grape	¼ cup
Orange	½ cup
Pineapple	⅓ cup
●—● Prune	¼ cup

Poached or baked fruit, fruit sorbet and fruit with a dash of liqueur can be used as desserts. Consider ½ cup as 1 serving.

FOOD CATEGORY 5: DAIRY PRODUCTS

Servings per day: 2 if low-fat or skim, 1 if whole-milk
Calories per serving: 80 for skim or low-fat milk, 160 for whole milk

Skim milk	1 cup
Buttermilk, skim	1 cup
Canned evaporated milk	½ cup
Cottage cheese, skim or low-fat; part-skim ricotta	½ cup
Cheese, part-skim mozzarella	1 ounce
Powdered (nonfat dry) milk	⅓ cup
Low-fat milk	1 cup
Yogurt, low-fat, nonfat flavored (vanilla, lemon, coffee)	¾ cup ½ cup

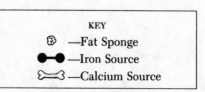

KEY
🍬 —Fat Sponge
●—● —Iron Source
⌇⊃ —Calcium Source

WHOLE-MILK PRODUCTS

Whole milk	1 cup
Buttermilk	1 cup
Canned, evaporated	½ cup
Cheese, hard aged or semisoft	1½ ounces
Yogurt, plain	1 cup
Ice cream*	1 small scoop

*consume only occasionally in place of all other fat *and* sugar

FOOD CATEGORY 6: FAT SOURCES

Servings per day: 3
Each serving provides 35–45 calories

Avocado	⅛ cup
Bacon, crisp	1 slice
Butter, margarine	1 tsp.
Chicken skin (Sometimes you've *got* to eat it!	1 (from breast)
Cream	
light	1 tbs.
heavy, sour	1 tbs.
Cream cheese	1 tbs.
French/ Italian dressing	3 tbs.
Mayonnaise	1 tsp.
Nuts	6 small
Oil or cooking fat	1 tsp.
Olives	5 small
Any oily-tasting or suspiciously creamy-looking sauce or dressing	1 tsp.

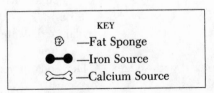

KEY
⊕ —Fat Sponge
●━● —Iron Source
⊂⊃ —Calcium Source

FOOD CATEGORY 7: SUGARS

Servings per day: 2 teaspoons sugar, jam, jelly or syrup
Calories per serving: 16

CONDIMENTS

You are free to dress up your food any way you like, as long as you use common sense. If a condiment or sauce is sweet or oily, it contains sugar or fat calories that must be accounted for. You can be a bit more liberal with sugary items such as sweet pickles than with oil-based items such as barbecue sauce. The items below on the left contain few or no calories, and may be used freely.

Use these *freely*:

Clear broth
Bouillon
Gelatin, unsweetened
Consommé
Dill, sour pickles
Pickled vegetables
Mustard
Soy sauce
Vinegar
Lemon, lime juice
Worcestershire sauce
All herbs and spices

Use these *rationally*:

Ketchup
Steak, barbecue sauce
Tomato sauce
Sweet relishes
Sweet pickles

BEVERAGES

Milk
Coffee
Tea
Water
Fruit juice mixed with seltzer
(watch calories)

Vegetable juice (watch calories)
Plain soda water with lemon or lime
Diet soda (if you absolutely must)

SNACK LIST

Snacks must, of course, fit into your daily calorie quota. If you don't have milk with lunch, for example, you can have it as a snack. If you haven't eaten much starch, you can have some crackers. Use common sense.

Fruit, dried or fresh
Milk shake (skim milk, nonfat milk powder, sugar, fruit or vanilla)
Popcorn—air-popped
Seeds
Whole-wheat crackers
Raw vegetables
Bouillon
Consommé
Dill pickles

SPLURGE LIST

You can select any *one* of the items below and add it to your menu every third day. Each provides about 100 calories. You may also substitute any splurge any day for your 100 calories of fat.

1 4-oz. glass red or white wine or champagne or 1½ oz. Scotch, gin, vodka, etc.
2 wine spritzers (made with ½ wine, ½ soda water)
1 *small* scoop ice cream
1½ ounces caviar
2 small chocolates
2 tablespoons chocolate syrup
2 filled cookies
1 ounce Brie, Camembert, etc., or cream cheese
1 tablespoon peanut butter
Any 100-calorie treat you crave!

THE BETTER BODY DIET MEAL SUGGESTIONS

I've found that rigid diet menus are hard to stick to for long because they don't allow for spontaneity, favorite dishes or eating out. While you can use the suggestions below successfully on your diet, you are not obligated to do so. They are simply guidelines for creating nutritious meals.

Suggested Breakfasts: about 300 calories

Note number of servings of each Food Category provided by meal suggestion.

Choose *one* item from each of the first two groups.

Bran muffin
2 slices whole-wheat toast
Bagel
Whole-wheat English muffin
2–3 whole-wheat pancakes
Any whole-grain cereal (1 oz.)

1 egg (poached; boiled; scrambled or fried in cooking spray, *or* low-cal omelet made with 3 whites, 1 yolk)
2 oz. canned salmon, tuna, sardines (packed in water, mustard, tomato sauce)
½ cup low-fat cottage cheese
1 ounce hard aged cheese
1 tablespoon peanut butter

> *plus:*

1 cup milk
1 citrus or other fruit or broiled tomato
Optional: 1 teaspoon of margarine/butter

Suggested Lunches (about 350 calories):

Note number of servings of each Food Category provided by meal suggestion.

Choose *one* item from the first group.

Large bowl of vegetable or any noncreamed homemade soup
  with bread or crackers
Split-pea soup with dark bread
Chicken or tuna-salad sandwich on whole-wheat bread
Meat or cheese sandwich on whole-wheat bread
Pita pizza (½ pita with tomato sauce, mozzarella)
Pita salad sandwich (cottage cheese, scallions, tomatoes, bean
  sprouts)
Large green salad with bread and cheese
Chef's salad, bread
1 cup plain yogurt, whole-wheat crackers, fruit
Cold pasta-and-vegetable salad
Fresh-fruit salad with cottage cheese or yogurt, whole-wheat
  crackers

> *plus:*

1 cup skim milk or plain yogurt
Optional: fruit, 1 teaspoon of butter/margarine/mayo

Suggested Dinners (about 500–600 calories):

Note number of servings of each Food Category provided
by meal suggestion.
Choose *one* item from the first group.

Spaghetti with meatballs
Lasagne
Chili
Hamburger
Lean steak
Macaroni and cheese
Roast chicken, whole-wheat bread stuffing
Soufflé
Cheese pizza with mushrooms and green peppers

Meat loaf (made with lean meat, whole-wheat bread)
Poached or baked chicken or fish
Beef or veal stew with vegetables
Baked pork chops
Liver and onions

plus:

One or more of the following:

Steamed vegetables (greens, broccoli, carrots)
Large green salad
Baked potato, yam
Marinated bean salad
Baked squash
Corn bread
Sautéed spinach and garlic
Cole slaw (oil/vinegar dressing)

RESTAURANT LUNCH, DINNER

You probably eat out fairly often. This list helps you do so safely. Be sure to make a guesstimate of how many servings of your allotted foods you're getting in a dish. For example, if you have a chicken taco with beans and rice, you're getting about three servings of starch (for the taco, beans and rice) and probably three servings of protein (for 2–3 ounces of chicken and the beans). Always ask what ingredients are in a particular dish. And never feel compelled to eat more than you want just because it's on your plate.

Fast food/Deli   Small plain burger, milk
Salad-bar salad (made of 1 scoop chick-peas or
    kidney bean salad, lots of greens, vinegar,
    dash of oil)

Meat or poultry sandwich (made of freshly
    sliced ham, turkey, corned beef, roast beef,
    etc.)
Sardine sandwich with mustard or tomato sauce
Tuna, salmon sandwich (made with whole can
    of fish, mustard, lettuce, tomato. You *cannot*
    control mayo in deli salads.)

French
Small slab of pâté with large green salad
Fish or chicken entrée with any *light* sauce
All aspics
All salads and vegetables
All uncreamed soups
All soufflés, with green salad
(Quiche is *not* low-fat or low-cal. Have only the
    tiniest sliver with a large green salad or soup.)

Japanese
Sashimi (raw fish) with rice
Sushi (raw fish wrapped around rice)
Sukiyaki (braised meat or poultry with vegeta-
    bles)
Broiled fish, chicken with rice

Chinese
Vegetable/shrimp/chicken chow mein, rice
All heavily vegetable, lightly sautéed dishes
    with rice
Broiled fish or seafood with vegetables

Mexican
Tacos, enchiladas, tostadas (chicken, beef,
    beans—no cheese, sour cream)
Beans and rice with tomato sauce
Chili

Spanish
Gazpacho
Paella with rice
All broiled or steamed seafood dishes with rice

BETTER FOOD PREPARATION TIPS:

• Measure out a level tablespoon and teaspoon each of mayonnaise, butter and cooking or salad oil. Memorize what these quantities of butter and mayo look like on the tip of a knife, on bread and on top of some tuna fish. Memorize what the oil looks like spread on the bottom of a frying pan and in a salad-dressing jar. Once you've done that, you'll never again go overboard.

• From now on, use no more than one teaspoon of oil in the vinaigrette on your salad. You don't need more than that.

• Note grams of fat per serving on food labels. Multiply by 9. That's how many calories of fat you're getting.

• Trim all visible fat from meat before cooking.

• Poach chicken or fish in wine (the calories evaporate) with herbs such as tarragon and dill.

• Broil, roast or braise meats instead of frying.

• Use cooking spray (no, it won't hurt you) whenever possible for frying. Eggs, hash browns and pancakes all taste fine without fat.

• When frying is unavoidable, start off food in cooking spray, and add a few drops of oil or butter for flavor in the last few minutes.

• Pat hamburgers and steaks with paper towels after cooking to blot up excess fat. You can remove 100 calories or more that way!

• Try making favorite recipes with half the oil called for. And always use good-quality oil—a little goes a long way.

• Refrigerate cooked stews and pot roasts overnight before serving. The fat will rise to the top and harden, making it easy to remove before reheating.

• Prepare marinated vegetable and bean salads in sweetened or rice vinegar, or lemon juice, without oil.

• Use lemon juice, spices and herbs on cooked vegetables instead of butter.

• Thicken gravy with pureed vegetables (carrots, leeks) cooked in sherry and broth instead of with fat and flour.

• Make more vegetable entrées, using meat as a side dish.

• Top potatoes with low-fat yogurt and chives rather than sour cream.

• Create creamy low-fat salad dressings out of cottage cheese, buttermilk or yogurt and herbs whirled in your blender.

• It *is* possible to wean yourself down to one sweet tooth instead of a full set. Just eliminate sugar gradually from coffee, fruit and anywhere you don't really need it.

• Try cutting sugar in pastry recipes in half by substituting fruit juices such as apple, orange, prune and pineapple. This also provides moisture, so it lets you cut down on fat too.

• Try using more sweet-tasting spices such as cloves, cinnamon, nutmeg and ginger in baked goods instead of so much sugar.

• Don't use so-called coffee whiteners—they are loaded with sugar and fat. Use evaporated low-fat or skim milk instead.

• Make high-calcium milk shakes out of skim or nonfat dry milk, vanilla or fruit and a bit of sugar or honey.

• Use whole-wheat all-purpose or pastry flour in baked goods such as brownies and for dredging meat or fish. If you don't mention it, your children won't know the difference.

• Keep sliced fresh vegetables in a bowl of ice water in the fridge for handy snacking.

• Look through Italian, Indian, Mexican and Spanish cookbooks for interesting ideas on how to serve vegetables as a main course. This automatically cuts down on calories.

• Make a habit of eating foods that must be peeled,

chewed a lot, cracked, or otherwise "worked for," such as oranges, artichokes and nuts and seeds in the shell. It's all too easy to down 500 fatty calories' worth of naked peanuts without realizing it. If a food is hard to get at, eating time is slowed down, and fewer calories are consumed. Also, eating is more fun and somehow more of a satisfying experience when you get to fondle and play with your food.

• Stock your desk at work with good things to nibble on, such as dried fruit, crackers, popcorn or seeds, so you won't have to resort to candy and cake or other empty-calorie "fat bombs" from the coffee wagon when you're hungry.

• The more you eat at one sitting, the more will be stored as fat. So become a nibbler—eat small meals more often, throughout the day. And don't save all your calories for a big dinner. Have something light during the day, so your body won't think it's fasting.

6 / The Better Body Shapers (Optional)

This chapter focuses on special things you can do for specific "problem" areas you'd like to firm up, smooth out and pare down. They are *not* a mandatory part of the Plan, however— *you only do the ones you need.* Without them, you'll still have a much better body at the end of six weeks, through Fat-Burning Sessions and the Better Body Diet alone. But if you do want sleeker upper arms, slimmer thighs and higher, more prominent breasts, the Better Body Shapers can provide them faster and more effectively than any so-called "spot reducers" you've ever tried.

I don't know about you, but I'm hopeless at floor exercises. Even a simple leg lift has always been beyond me. After one or two feeble lurches, the leg in question would begin quivering, a condition which escalated into spasms that would soon rack the rest of my body, whereupon I would invariably flop over, cracking my ankle on the coffee table.

Besides the excruciating pain and embarrassing lack of grace that invariably accompany their execution, floor exercises are fraught with problems for the average lazy person. In order for those torturous exertions to work, you have to do a lot of different ones, you have to do them religiously and—

the most critical variable of all—you have to do them *right*. Unfortunately, correct form invariably requires a degree of flexibility found only in prepubescent Rumanian gymnasts.

Flexibility is an important part of general fitness. But it is not your first priority in achieving a better body, since the act of getting flexible—say, during yoga—does not burn fat or give one a zippier metabolism. (And flexibility is invisible. Nobody ever complimented me on my flexibility—at least not on the first date.) So you'll be relieved to know that you'll never again have to spend painful hours agonizingly spread-eagled on the carpet. To attain total tautness of any flabby body area fast, you need only spend 2–3 minutes a day doing the best and easiest muscle shaper of all: weight lifting.

"*Weight* Lifting? You *must* be kidding!"

No. But the kind of weight lifting we're talking about here doesn't involve grunting and groaning under huge barbells. Nor does it turn you into a musclebound body builder. You have to work terribly hard to look like that. And since you're a woman, you can't easily build the kind of "bulk" you see on men. That's due to the male hormone testosterone, of which most women have *very* little. Your Body Shapers start you off with very light weights, which are all you ever need to firm you up and trim inches. You can do many of the Better Body Shapers sitting on or even lying down on your bed watching TV. And since you work only one muscle group at a time, you don't get exhausted. They are truly the perfect lazy way to banish jiggles and droops anywhere on your body—and increase your joint flexibility at the same time.

HOW YOUR BETTER BODY SHAPERS WORK

While it is easy to "cheat" at calisthenics by doing them halfheartedly and thereby underworking many muscles at once, weight lifting allows you to isolate an individual muscle or muscle group and overload it sufficiently so that it is stimulated to develop to its maximum potential. Just two weeks of working with weights can accomplish more than *months* of floor exercises. Best of all, the Body Shapers don't *hurt*, because they don't demand that you crunch your body into a position that wasn't intended by nature.

No localized exercise can remove the layer of fat directly above any one muscle. That's the job of your Fat-Burning Sessions and your Better Body Diet. But while you're busy achieving your general fat loss, the Better Body Shapers will be making *muscles* in key body "problem areas" much firmer and more compact, so that they take up less space. That means you can lose inches wherever you want. Once muscles are slimmer and firmer—the first step in body shaping—and you then want to add inches anywhere, you simply need to increase the weight you use.

A bonus you get for doing all the Better Body Shapers as suggested is that you will very probably more than *double* your strength in six weeks. This is also important to a better body, because a stronger body stands taller and is less prone to injury. You may not want to be an Amazon, but you do want to have enough muscle power to lift your growing child or your luggage without strain. And besides, it's a great feeling knowing you've got it when you need it.

If you are close to your "ideal" (but still overfat) weight, you will probably notice a sizable loss of inches in areas you shape in the third week of the Plan. If you need to lose a lot of weight, your muscles are currently covered by more fat, so you may not see such dramatic results right away. But your flesh will soon begin to look much firmer and tighter. The muscles will continue to shape up inside you, and as you continue losing fat, you will gradually begin to see splendid new contours.

Your Better Body Shapers can also go a long way toward reversing the effects of repeated weight gain and loss, which may have left your skin stretched. Firm muscle can help fill in the empty spaces where shapeless fat used to be. This helps make stretch marks much less noticeable.

Best of all, a well-muscled body can afford to carry *more* fat. Remember the times when you dieted yourself down to a stick? Your thighs looked skinny, but your breasts all but disappeared, and your face looked gaunt. When you build more muscle all over, you can carry a slightly higher level of fat on top of them, which allows you to have firm thighs and *still* keep your bosom and your cheeks.

GETTING STARTED

In order to develop each muscle fully during your Better Body Shapers, as much of the muscle must be doing the work as possible so that maximum growth occurs. To accomplish this, it's important to move the muscle through the entire range of motion of the joint to which it's attached. For example, to correctly develop your biceps muscle, you hold a weight in your hand and fully extend your lower arm downward, then bring it upward, opening and closing your elbow joint as far as it will go. By doing this, you are also improving your joint flexibility without really trying.

One complete movement (such as the aforementioned opening and closing of your arm) is called a repetition—or, in official iron-pumping lingo, a "rep." A collection of reps is called a "set." Your muscle firms up best if you do at least 8–12 reps per set. After doing one set, you may rest *briefly*—meaning less than 1 minute—then do another set. (If you rest longer between sets, your muscle has a chance to recover from the effort, and this lessens the muscle-shaping potential of the exercise.) Many repetitions with a light weight tend to slenderize and firm a muscle, which results in the loss of inches. This is what will happen at first in all body areas, because your muscles are currently flabby. After maximum firmness is achieved, then additional shaping and adding of inches can begin, if that's what you desire—for example, on your chest and shoulders. To accomplish this, you simply use heavier weights.

Maximum development of a muscle cannot happen if an exercise is done too quickly. So be sure to do each complete repetition in a slow, fluid motion (no jerking) taking at least 4–6 seconds.

You will get the best and quickest results if you do your chosen Better Body Shapers three times a week for the suggested number of reps and sets. For the first time out, do as many reps as you can, just to get the hang of it. From then on you can do each Shaper as instructed, or do as many reps and sets as you want beyond the minimum.

You can also increase the weight as indicated whenever you are ready. Progressing to a new weight usually takes two weeks, but you can do so whenever the weight feels too light and the effort is too easy.

You can do your Better Body Shapers almost anytime— right after a Fat-Burning Session, if you wish. (Don't do leg exercises before your Session, however, or your legs will have less glucose than they need to make your fat burn.) You may scatter different Shapers throughout the day, or do them all at once.

WHAT TO WEAR

You may wear anything that's comfortable and allows free movement of your limbs. A T-shirt and shorts are fine. A leotard is nice because it lets you see how you're shaping up both during your workout—you can watch your muscles temporarily grow bigger as they get "pumped up" with blood—and from workout to workout; and because a leotard and tights tend to smooth out fat. Or you can wear my standard outfit, nothing, which is definitely convenient and a touch primal.

THE RIGHT EQUIPMENT

To start with, you will need:

one set of two 2½-pound wrist/ankle weights
one set of two 5-pound wrist/ankle weights

and:
one set of two 2½-pound dumbbells
one set of two 5-pound dumbbells

or:
Space Weights®

or:
2 small detergent or bleach bottles filled with water, sand or dirt; or sugar boxes, or full juice cans, or iron pots or pans

Wrist/ankle weights can be used on arms or legs. They can be worn around your ankles during rebound jogging sessions, or strapped together to make a weight belt to wear while you're walking. You can also increase the weight you use for upper-body Shapers by wearing a wrist weight in addition to holding a dumbbell. (For example, to increase the weight from 5 to 7½ pounds, you would wear a 2½-pound wrist weight and hold a 5-pound dumbbell.)

Dumbbells (which, by the way, are called that because some look like bells but are mute—not because they are used by brainless jocks) don't come only in black iron. They are now made of water- or sand-filled plastic and come in many pretty colors, costing about $10–$15 a pair. Chrome weights, though elegant, cost about $25 a pair.

I especially like a versatile new type of football-shaped weights called Space Weights®. They can be filled with water, sand, wet sand or lead shot, depending on the weight you need. They have hollowed-out grips which allow them to be used in your hands or, for some leg exercises, on your feet. They cost about $25 a pair. If you can't find them in your local sporting-goods store, call the Grayfar Corporation, 1 (313) 862-9195, for shopping information.

While you should get wrist/ankle weights (you can't pick up a dumbbell with your toes), you don't have to buy dumbbells. You can instead use detergent or bleach bottles with large openings at the handle filled with the correct weight of water, sand or dirt. You can also use boxes of sugar, which already come in convenient weights, full cans of juice or even iron pots and pans, which have convenient handles.

NO MORE JELLY LEGS

Even if you don't seem flabby anywhere else, you are probably, like most women, unhappy with the state of your thighs. You may have the dimpling that some call "cellulite." Or you may have flabby inner thighs, or "saddlebags" at your sides. Your Fat-Burning Sessions will go a long way toward solving these problems, because along with removing fat, they firm muscles too. But if you need a bit more reshaping anywhere, there is a Better Body Shaper to help you. If you just want all-around firming, the Total Thigh Shaper will give you all you need. You will definitely notice firming and see new contours within two weeks.

THIGH SHAPER SERIES

General instructions: Start with 2½-pound ankle weights. Do 2 sets of 15 reps of each Thigh Shaper you need. After two weeks add at least 1 more set. Increase the weight to 5, 7½, then 10 pounds when weight becomes too easy, and if you desire more shaping beyond firmness.

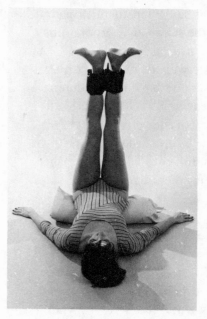

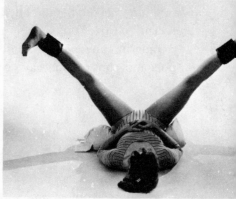

Inner-Thigh Shaper

Starting position: With weights on ankles, lie face up on bed or floor, placing rolled towel under hips for support. Raise legs together toward ceiling with toes pointed outward and feet flat, as if walking like Charlie Chaplin.

Slowly open legs as wide as possible, then slowly close, leading with your heels. Repeat as directed.

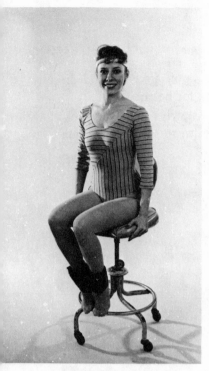
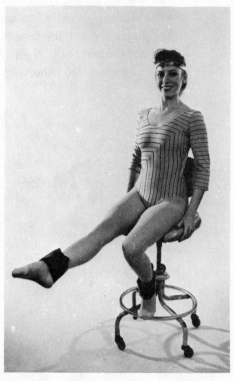

Front Thigh Shaper

Starting position: With weights on ankles, sit on edge of high chair with legs together, knees bent, and back straight. Grip sides of chair for balance.

Extend one leg straight out. Hold briefly, and return to starting position. Repeat as directed. Do other leg.

Outer-Thigh/ Buttock/ Hip Shaper

Starting position: With weights on ankles, stand directly behind chair, holding on to back for balance.

Keeping back and leg straight, slowly extend leg back at an angle away from body, then return to starting position. Repeat as directed. Do other leg.

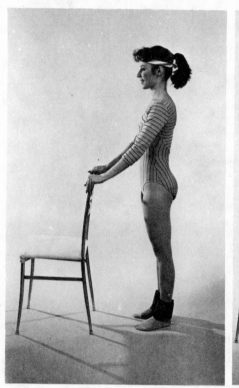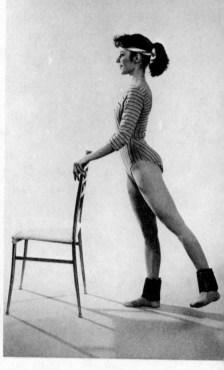

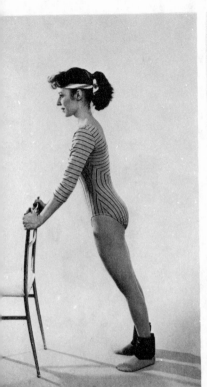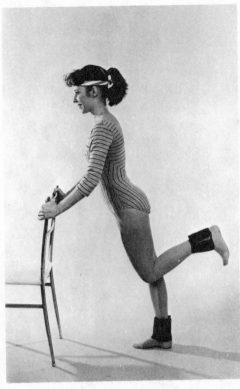

Back Thigh Shaper

Starting position: With weights on ankles, stand 1½ feet behind chair, holding on for balance, and tilt body forward in a straight line.

Kick one leg back slowly from knee, keeping upper leg straight from hip. Return to starting position. Repeat as directed. Do other leg.

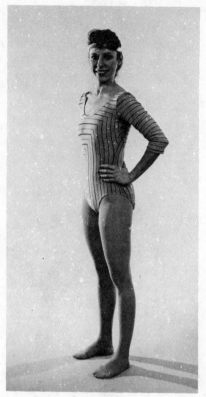
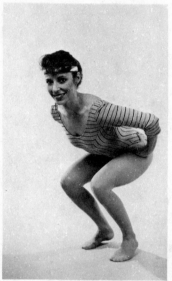

Total Thigh Shaper

No weight needed.

Starting position: Stand with feet slightly apart, back straight, hands resting lightly on hips.

Slowly bend knees until thighs are parallel (or nearly parallel) to the floor, keeping heels down as far as you can; in other words, squat. (Your upper body will lean forward, but your back should be straight, not hunched over.) Return slowly to standing position. Repeat as directed, and increase to as many as you can do.

A WELL-TURNED CALF

If you have flat feet, as I do, you may also have a flat inner calf, as I once did. This Shaper will give you a shapelier all-around calf, and a sleeker ankle too.

Calf Shaper

No weight needed.

Starting position: Stand on balls of feet on edge of step or on unbound edge of thick book, with toes pointing straight ahead. (If you want to build up inner calf muscle, point toes slightly outward.)

Raise body up on toes, then slowly lower yourself as far down as possible, so you feel a stretch in your Achilles tendon. Do *not* bounce. Do as many reps as you can, but work up to at least 25. Add ankle weights, if you wish, after two weeks.

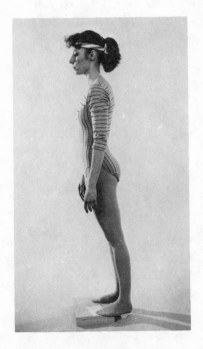 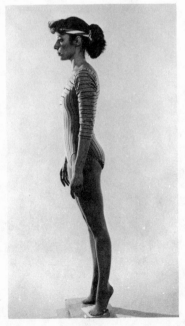

A STRONG STOMACH

You've got that extra layer of fat to get rid of. But you've also got weak abdominal muscles and, most likely, bad posture, which is also caused mostly by weak abdominal muscles. Perhaps you have had a baby—or several. Put it all together and you have a bulge you've been battling for years, always in vain.

The best, most efficient way to tighten those muscles fast is with sit-ups. But we're not talking here about the kind that make you flop back and forth like a demented rag doll. Those don't work your abdominal muscles properly, and can even throw your back out.

The special lazy sit-ups you'll be doing don't require you to sit up all the way. What they do is make you use your upper body as a weight, which is lifted by the entire abdominal region from your rib cage to your pubic bone. I've found they work better than anything else. They may not give you the concave abdomen of your (or someone else's) youth. But they

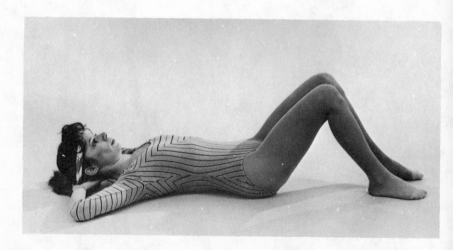

will give you the smallest, firmest stomach it's possible for *you* to have.

Stomach Shaper

No weight needed.

Starting position: Lie on back on floor, with knees bent, feet flat on floor. Place hands behind neck.

Keeping small of your back on floor, slowly *curl* spine forward so your elbows are almost facing foward. Only your head and neck should leave the floor, *not* your back. Hold 3–4 seconds, then slowly lower body to starting position. Contract and flatten abdominal muscles throughout entire rep, so they are doing the work, not your back muscles. Do 15 reps, at least three times per week. After two weeks, do 25 reps three times per week. At first you may be able to do only 5 repetitions. That's okay. Just keep adding reps each time you try it, so that by the third try you can do 15, and by the end of the second week you can do 25.

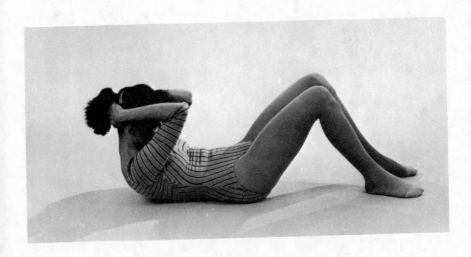

WAIST AWAY

Some call them love handles. Some call them belly rolls. Whatever your pet name for them, they are the handfuls of flesh you can grab at either side of your waist. Part of that is fat you will be losing, but some of the slackness is due to poor muscle tone underneath. This Waist Shaper will tighten those muscles and trim inches off your waist.

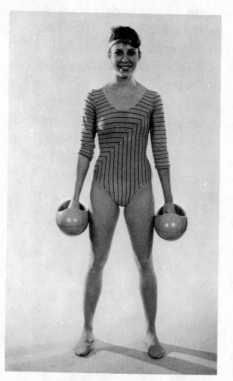 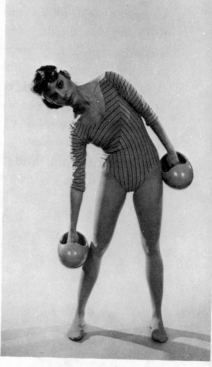

Waist Shaper

Start with two 5-pound dumbbells.

Starting position: Holding dumbbells straight down at your sides in overhand grip, stand with feet apart and back straight.

Slowly lean from the waist to one side as far as you can without bending forward or backward. Then lean to the other side as far as you can go. Do 2 sets of 10 reps in each direction. After two weeks, add at least 1 more set. Increase weight to 7½, then 10 pounds when previous weight becomes too easy.

BREASTS THAT CAN RATE A "10"

The one area of your body you may want to add inches to—or at least, not *lose* any from—is your chest. You may have too much of a good thing, or what you think is not enough. Whatever your natural endowments, you naturally want to make the most of them.

Since breast tissue is composed primarily of fat and glands, you can increase the size of breasts themselves only by gaining weight, having an implant, getting pregnant or taking the Pill. Your genetic makeup—i.e., how your fat is distributed—determines how general weight loss will affect your breast size.

Regardless of how much actual breast tissue you have, however, the state of your pectoral muscles—those muscles underlying the breasts—has a great deal to do with how outstanding your breasts are. Poor pectoral muscle tone makes even the perkiest breasts pout, large breasts sag and smaller breasts look much flatter. A sunken-looking breastbone above even nicely rounded breasts is also a common unflattering problem. If you want a higher, younger look, and cleavage that naturally coaxes the eye to the architectural wonders adjacent, you can build it with weights no matter what your actual breast size—just as many models do.

The classic chest builder, which you have often seen weight lifters do, is the "bench press," so named because the lifter usually does it lying face up on a bench and pushes, or presses, the barbell or dumbbells straight up over his chest and back again. It is a good all-around firmer of the pectoral muscles for both sexes, and can be done on the floor as well as on a bench or bed. Each of the Shapers illustrated below gives as good a general firming-up of the pectorals as the bench press, but each also has a special breast-molding function. The Cleavage Maker, which builds the middle pectorals, can create impressive contours you never had before, and—yes—can actually add inches to your chest. The Breastbone Filler adds a slope above that makes breasts look much fuller. The Breast Lifter gives breasts the support they need against gravity, and makes smaller breasts much more prominent.

You will see results within two weeks. The more Shapers you do, of course, and the more faithfully you do them, the more spectacular those results will be.

BREAST SHAPER SERIES

General Instructions: Start with two 2½-pound dumbbells. Do 2 sets of 10 reps of each Shaper you need. After two weeks, add at least 1 more set. Increase weight to 5, 7½, then 10 pounds when previous weight becomes too easy.

Cleavage Maker

Starting position: Holding dumbbells in underhand grip, lie on floor or diagonally on bed with head at one corner. Extend arms outward from sides, with elbows slightly bent.

Slowly bring arms together above you. Lower slowly to starting position. Repeat as directed.

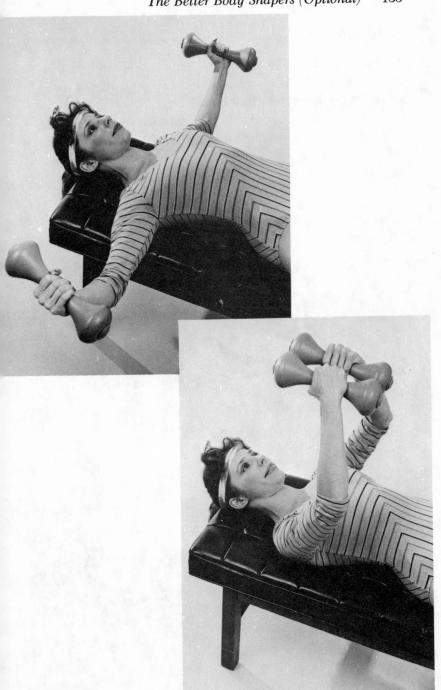

Breast Lifter

Starting position: Holding dumbbells in overhand grip, lie on floor or diagonally on bed with head at one corner. Extend arms straight back over your head.

Keeping elbows locked, lift arms forward in an arch over chest, palms facing each other, until arms almost touch your sides. Hold briefly, then slowly return to starting position. Repeat as directed.

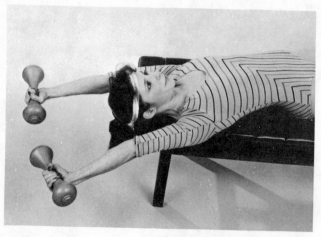

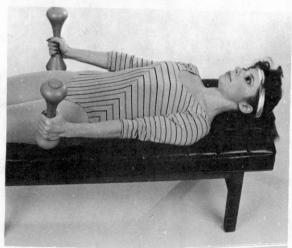

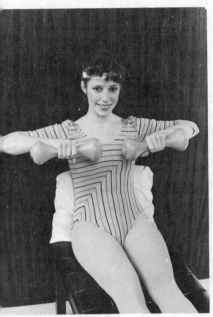 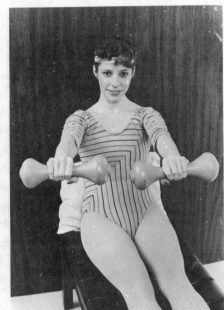

Breastbone Filler

Starting position: Lie with legs outstretched on couch or bed, leaning your back against armrest or wall at 45-degree angle. Support back with pillow. Holding dumbbells in overhand grip, lift arms, elbows bent inward so that weights are at chest level.

Slowly extend arms straight out in front of you, parallel to legs. Hold briefly, then bring weights back to chest. Repeat as directed.

HOW TO BE WELL ARMED

You may have two major unsightly problems on your upper arms: lumpy pads of storage fat on the outside that bulge when your arm is at your side, and a small slack muscle that becomes a wobbly curve underneath when your arm is outstretched.

These conditions are not inevitable with age. Although overstretched skin from excessive weight loss may contribute to the saggy look, the most important factors are too much fat and underdeveloped triceps muscles. Since the triceps muscles are notoriously underused in women, yours are very likely quite weak at this point. So you'll be starting with a very low weight. If 2½ pounds is too heavy, use a 1-pound box of sugar until you're stronger.

The contracted biceps muscle is, of course, the one men perennially proffer for admiration and fondling; frankly, I get a kick out of flexing mine these days! You don't want to have a baseball sitting on your arm—but you don't want a limp rubber band, either. Underdeveloped biceps combined with shriveled triceps—both covered in fat—add up to arms that resemble two pink sausages about to burst out of their casings.

Your biceps aren't quite as underdeveloped as your triceps, since they are the main muscle involved in carrying whatever you usually carry. So you will be using a heavier weight to start.

Triceps Shaper

Start with two 2½-pound dumbbells.

Starting position: Standing with legs slightly apart and knees slightly bent, bend forward from the hips until torso is

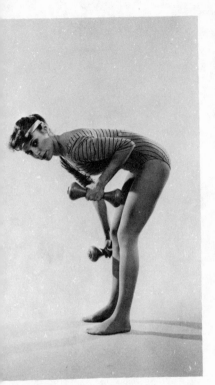 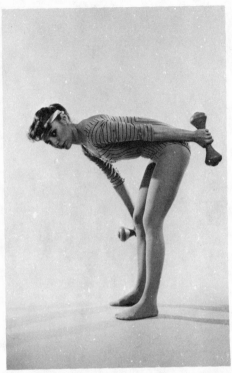

parallel to floor. Holding dumbbells in an overhand grip, raise one weight near to chest, elbow tightly at your side.

Extend forearm back as if doing slow karate chop, keeping upper arm glued to your side. Bring weight back to chest. Do 2 sets of 10 reps with each arm. After two weeks, add at least 1 more set. Increase weight to 5, 7½, then 10 pounds when previous weight becomes too easy. This Shaper can also be done while kneeling near edge of sofa or bed.

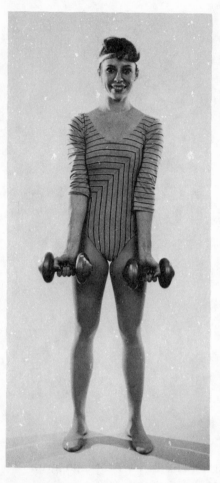 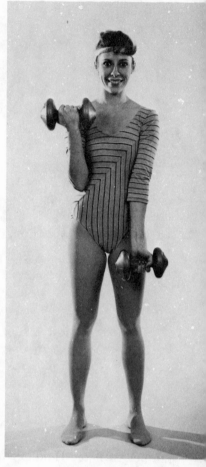

Biceps Shaper

Start with two 5-pound dumbbells.

Starting position: Stand with legs slightly apart and back straight, holding dumbbells straight down in front of you in an underhand grip.

Slowly lift one dumbbell to chest, bending only your elbow and keeping upper arm stationary and back straight. Do not jerk weight. Slowly lower. Do 2 sets of 10 reps with each arm. Increase weight to 7½, then 10 pounds when previous weight becomes too easy. This Shaper may also be done sitting on edge of sofa with your elbow on your knee; lean forward and use other hand to brace working arm.

A BEAUTIFUL BACK

Bad posture and backaches are both due primarily to weak back muscles. Banishing both is remarkably easy. The following Back Shapers give you a stronger, straighter back—one far less likely to get "thrown out"—along with gentle, sexy ripples. It's best to do all of them as a series in succession.

Note: If you have a diagnosed back injury or ailment, you must consult your doctor before doing these Shapers.

BACK SHAPER SERIES

General Instructions: Start with two 2½-pound dumbbells. Do 1 set each of 15 repetitions. After two weeks, add at least 1 more set. Increase weight to 5, 7½, then 10 pounds when previous weight becomes too easy.

Lower-Back Shaper

Starting position: Stand with feet apart, knees locked, holding dumbbells straight down in front of you in overhand grip.

Bend slowly forward from waist, and try to touch dumbbells to floor. Slowly stand upright. Do not jerk up and down. Repeat as directed. (As you know, you are not supposed to lift a *heavy* weight this way; you are supposed to bend your knees and lift with your legs. But using weights as described is the correct way to strengthen those notoriously weak lower-back muscles so your back will be better protected from injury, aches and fatigue in the future.)

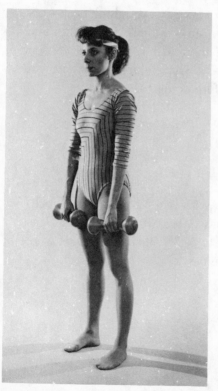
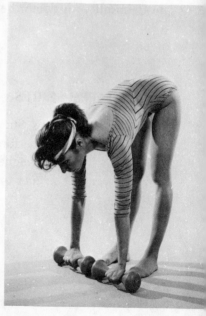

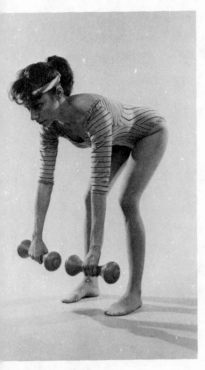 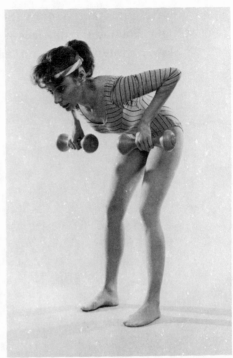

Middle-Back Shaper

Starting position: Standing with legs apart and knees slightly bent, bend forward so chest is parallel to floor. Holding dumbbells in overhand grip, extend arms toward floor with palms facing knees.

Slowly pull weights toward chest, bending elbows, then extend again, as if rowing a boat. Repeat as directed.

Upper-Back Shaper

Starting position: Stand with legs slightly apart and back straight, holding dumbbells at sides in overhand grip.

Slowly shrug shoulders up and down. Repeat as directed.

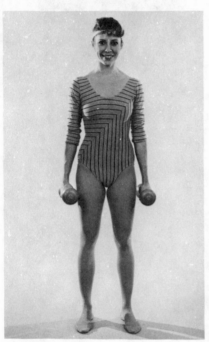 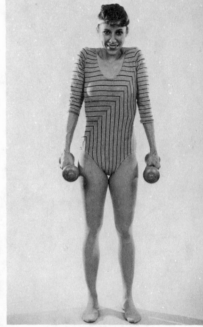

SAGGING SHOULDERS

If your body has a pear-shaped look, the problem may not be unusually big hips or a large waist, but narrow shoulders due to underdeveloped deltoid muscles. Shaping up this neglected area is one of the most dramatic ways you can alter the visual proportions of your whole body. These Shapers will give you rounder, sexier and stronger shoulders you will be proud to display in bare tops.

SHOULDER SERIES

General Instructions: Start with two 2½-pound dumbbells. Do 2 sets each of 10 reps (or as many repetitions as you can). After two weeks, add at least 1 more set. Increase weight to 5, 7½, then 10 pounds when previous weight becomes too easy.

Front Shoulder Shaper

Starting position: Stand with feet slightly apart, back straight, holding dumbbells straight down in front of you in overhand grip.

With elbows locked, slowly raise arms until they are over your head. Lower slowly to starting position. Repeat as directed.

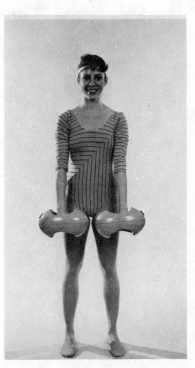
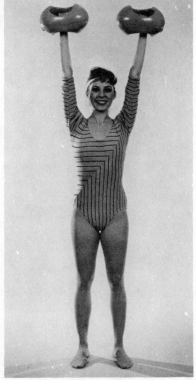

Top Shoulder Shaper

Starting position: Stand with feet slightly apart, back straight, holding dumbbells straight down at your sides in overhand grip.

With elbows bent and palms facing down, slowly raise arms away from your sides until weights are at shoulder level. Slowly lower to starting position. Repeat as directed.

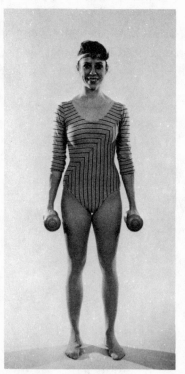 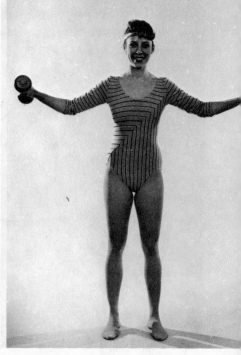

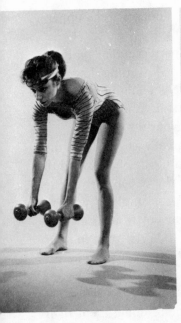
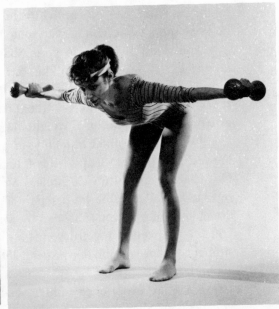

Back Shoulder Shaper

Starting position: Standing with feet slightly apart and knees slightly bent, bend forward from hips until chest is parallel to floor. Hold dumbbells straight down in overhand grip, your palms facing each other.

With elbows locked, slowly raise arms to shoulder height, then slowly lower, as if flapping your wings. Repeat as directed.

LAZY SHAPING TIPS

• Keep your weights at hand, so you don't have to go hunting for them. Stash a set of dumbbells and leg weights under your bed so you can, for example, do your breast and inner thigh Shapers when you wake up. Put another set under your sofa, so you can whip them out for some upper-body Shapers while you're watching TV.

• You don't have to do your Shapers standing or lying down. Do them while walking around waiting for your morning coffee to brew—a good way to get your blood going. If you have a private office, do them during your coffee break at work. Just keep a set of weights in your desk drawer.

• Fight your instinct to hold your breath when you do the hardest part of your Shaper (the actual lifting of the weight). Do what weight lifters do: inhale on the easier part of the rep, and exhale on the harder part. For example, if you are doing your biceps, you *in*hale on the way down, and *ex*hale as you lift the weight toward your chest. Do not suck *in* your stomach when you inhale; instead, let your entire abdomen expand.

• You may experience mild soreness after the first time you do your Shapers. That's a sign you're doing them *right* and that your muscles are getting enough stimulation to grow. Take a warm bath. If you are so sore the next day that you can't move, however, you are overdoing it. Lower the weight or the number of repetitions until you are sufficiently conditioned. It's also best to skip a day between workouts to give muscles time to repair themselves and build new tissue.

• Doing all the upper-body Shapers will make your top half look gorgeous and youthful. If you choose to do so, do them in this order: chest, lower back, middle back, upper back, shoulders, waist, triceps, biceps and stomach. The whole sequence takes less than 15 minutes. If you do all the lower-body Shapers, do them in this order: inner thighs, front thighs, back thighs, hips, buttocks, total thighs and calves. All of these should take you less than 15 minutes.

7 / Special Help for Special Needs

FATIGUE

Fatigue is a Catch-22–type problem that seems insurmountable. How can you even contemplate exercising when you don't have any energy to begin with?

Barring medical causes, the reason you feel so tired all the time is that you are so out of condition. Being sedentary actually *causes* fatigue. Your body isn't in shape to meet the demands of ordinary living, much less stressful situations. All your energy-release systems are depressed. This is *not* a normal state for the human body to be in.

It may seem that running a house or an office—or both—gives you all the exercise you need. Your days may be hectic. But the constant low-level activity—occasionally interspersed with strenuous tasks—that you perform while doing housework only wears you out. Of course, sitting at a desk all day is even worse.

Without regular fat-burning activity, your capacity to do even your ordinary tasks deteriorates. You get more and more tired. You *must* have that periodic muscle and cardiovascular overload to stay in condition. Once you begin waking up your metabolism and strengthening your major muscle groups, you will be able to breeze through the busiest day with energy to spare.

When you're feeling mentally wrung out, a Fat-Burning Session may be just what the doctor ordered. In fact, some psychiatrists now prescribe exercise for their patients instead of drugs, because it acts as a natural tranquilizer, banishing tension and depression. Instead of having a drink when you get home from work, have a Fat-Burning Session. It could provide all the relaxation you need. Then if you still want that drink, it's okay—you've already burned it off!

If after starting the Plan you are still constantly tired, you should, of course, see your doctor for a complete physical, including blood tests, to check whether or not you are anemic.

YOU'VE GOT A LOT TO LOSE

I won't lie to you.

If you have been overweight most of your life, or are now more than 50 pounds overweight, you simply can't lose it all in six weeks. Achieving a truly better body may take a few months—or much longer. But consider how long you have been struggling unsuccessfully with your weight. If you put all the diets you've tried end to end, you'd probably discover you've already spent far more than a year of your life so far getting nowhere! Now, at last, there is something that can really help you achieve your elusive goal. And there's no rush. Now that you are finally on the right track, you have all the time in the world.

Because you have been overfat for so long, you do have a major renovation in store. You have underdeveloped muscles. Your metabolism is unquestionably low. These are the very problems that the Plan is designed to correct. And it also allows you to do so safely and at your own speed.

Because you have been sedentary for most or all of your life, you need a fat-burning activity that isn't too strenuous. Your weight may even have caused you some joint problems. You may currently find even walking more than a few blocks hard on your hips, knees or feet. The stationary bicycle is the ideal fat-burning aid for you, because it takes your weight off your joints while simultaneously strengthening them and the muscles that support them. And it protects your privacy.

It's very wise to do as many Better Body Shapers as you can manage. By building up all your major muscles, you will minimize the sagging of skin as you lose your fat. If you are very well padded right now, you may not see the results of your efforts in six weeks. But your muscles *will* continue to develop invisibly. And you will be able to *feel* a new firmness almost right away. As the fat disappears, a whole new firm body will begin to emerge, rather than simply a skinnier but still flabby body.

One of the characteristics of overweight eating habits is "automatic" eating. You may eat simply because it's lunchtime, because the food smells good or because you're at a party. These are *external* cues. What the Better Body Diet will help you do is rediscover your internal appetite signals and your actual biological hunger. What's more, you will not have to desperately wait until mealtime if you're hungry, because you can eat certain foods as often as you need to. Since you will be choosing your food on merit as well as taste, you will, of course, have to be more discriminating than in the past. Admit it—you have lousy eating habits! No matter how overfat you are, you could very well be deficient in many nutrients, because you have probably been neglecting your nutritional needs. So read the nutritional information in Chapter 5 carefully.

You can stay on the 1200-calorie Better Body Diet as long

as you want, because it is a completely balanced and health-ful way to diet. But it's okay if you'd like to stop dieting for two weeks or so every few months, as long as you don't go wild *and you keep doing your Fat-Burning Sessions.* The best and healthiest way to relax your diet while continuing to lose weight (though more slowly) is to eat the minimum number of calories you would eat to maintain your "ideal" weight—a number you arrive at by multiplying your goal weight by 12. You must choose the extra calories from starches, vegetables and fruits—not fudge! Do watch fat intake, because it turns to body fat so easily. One small piece of cheesecake or any fa-vorite treat won't hurt now and then, however, and will pre-vent you from feeling deprived.

While following the Plan, you'll probably lose weight quite rapidly at first. That's because you may have been re-taining extra water. Also, the number of calories you'll be taking in to lose your fat may initially be dramatically lower than that which you would require to maintain your current weight, so you'll lose fat fast too. As you reach a lower and lower weight and the calories on the diet more closely ap-proach the calories you'll eventually need to maintain your target weight, your weight loss will slow down. Precisely how much weight you will lose over the coming months depends on how overfat you are now, and the magnitude of the meta-bolic problem you currently may have. But you can expect to lose *at least* a pound a week. In any case, unless you have a very slow metabolism (which may be the case owing to chronic inactivity), you will almost assuredly lose a lot more than 10 pounds of fat in six weeks.

Most important of all, you *must* be patient with yourself. The many changes that must take place to transform yours into a better body take time. You can always lose weight on a quickie diet—but you can't win a new and permanently "leaner" metabolism that way.

THE PREGNANT AMAZON

If you become pregnant while on the Plan, you *must* eat the way your doctor recommends. Now is not the time to diet. But there's no reason to stop doing your Fat-Burning Sessions and your Better Body Shapers. In fact, they are the best possible things you can do to prepare for that most strenuous of athletic events, childbirth.

Recent medical studies show that women who exercise regularly have far shorter labor, and less painful or pain-free deliveries. Some women who had been unfit during previous pregnancies report that their postfitness babies literally "popped out," whereas their other deliveries were difficult. Most importantly, a mother's exercise has not been shown to have any ill effects on her infant.

For these reasons, more and more physicians now feel exercise is essential for the pregnant, or about-to-be pregnant, woman. If you are already pregnant, you should not do any kind of exercise without first getting the go-ahead from your doctor. For the first three months you may be too nauseated to do anything anyway. But from then on, you can do whatever you feel like doing—even up to the day of delivery.

Your most critical priority is aerobic conditioning, produced by your fat-burning activity. It will help you get through the coming months with more energy, and give you the strength and stamina you'll need for the delivery.

You may do Fat-Burning Sessions exactly as described. Using a stationary bike is a very good idea because it takes the weight off your feet and back. If four 30-minute Sessions seem a bit much, at least consider taking a brief walk, 15 minutes or so, every day. This may make you excessively tired at first. Fine—go home and take a nap. But even that 15-minute walk will greatly improve your fitness.

Building endurance isn't the only important effect of

biking or walking. Many pregnant women experience water retention, especially in their legs, and develop varicose veins for the first time. Moving your legs regularly greatly improves circulation, which prevents the fluid buildup and the pooling of blood that contributes to puffy ankles and varicose veins.

As a baby continues to grow heavier, its weight places an increasing strain on your spine. In an attempt to compensate and balance yourself you may pull your pelvis backward, and develop a swayback. This very often causes pain, because weak and underdeveloped back muscles are so common today. If you have no back problems (other than ordinary aches) and can still bend over comfortably, you should be sure to do the Back Shapers in Chapter 6. They will also prepare you to do all the lifting and carrying you will have to do when the baby arrives.

Doing the Waist and Stomach Shapers will help you have the muscle power you need to push when the time comes—and will give you a head start on bringing your abdomen back to normal after the delivery.

Your breasts, of course, will swell over the coming months. Whether or not you choose to breast-feed, doing the Breast Shapers in Chapter 6 can help ward off possible sagging. Building up the pectoral muscles will have no effect on your ability to nurse your baby. You can even continue to do the exercises throughout lactation, if you wish.

After the Baby Comes

If you are fit, you will bounce back from the birth much faster. Whether you may diet or not depends on whether or not you are nursing. But if your doctor says okay, you can start exercising again within two weeks. Just start *gradually*.

But what if you haven't kept in shape during your pregnancy? Now you are many pounds overweight, and most of it seems to be located in your abdomen. With an infant keeping you up until all hours, you haven't a moment to yourself. All you really want is three solid weeks of uninterrupted sleep.

It may seem like the ultimate in absurdity, but the best cure for your condition is fat-burning activity. It will be very hard to get motivated at first. You may have to wait at least two months, until you and your baby fall into some kind of pattern. But once you get going, you will soon begin to feel mentally as well as physically more capable of handling the demands of new-motherhood.

The best fat-burning activity for you is probably stationary cycling, because you can pedal while the baby naps—even if for only 15 minutes at a time. Do *only* what you feel capable of doing. But after just a few Sessions, you *will* begin to feel better.

If you are nursing your baby, you must of course follow the diet that your doctor prescribes. But milk production consumes huge quantities of calories—at least 1000 a day—and most women find they lose weight spontaneously even while eating larger amounts of food than they normally do. So you may see the pounds drop off without even dieting! Fat-Burning Sessions will, of course, greatly speed this loss.

Whether you are nursing or not, your baby would much rather be tended by a mother who is relaxed, energetic, happy and able to cope than by one who is constantly exhausted, tense, angry and disgusted with her body. In order to become that kind of mother, you should not feel guilty about hiring a sitter from time to time so you can have an hour or two to spend on yourself.

FORTY AND BEYOND: IT'S NEVER TOO LATE

You're not a kid anymore. The prospect of renovating your thighs seems mighty dim. And you've been losing weight just by dieting since you were a teenager, so you probably don't have much muscle left anyway. The only thing that might help now is an entire body transplant. Why beat a dead horse?

It's not time to give up—it's time to *get* up! Many recent studies have shown that the most effective way to improve one's health and physical condition at any age is to perform regular fat-burning activity. Many of the so-called symptoms of aging—such as a shift toward a fatter body composition, loss of lean muscle tissue, decrease in bone density and strength, loss of vitality and one's sex drive, and even senility—are now known to be worsened or caused by sedentary living. If there are 80-year-olds who run in marathons—and there are quite a few—surely you can get your body going too!

Increasing stiffness of joints does come with age, and can be quite disabling—if you let it. Fat-Burning Sessions and Better Body Shapers both have a rejuvenating effect on the tendons and ligaments, stimulating growth and making connective tissues stronger, more pliant and less apt to be injured. You can restore a truly amazing degree of flexibility to your body simply by moving around regularly.

Sedentary people tend to get even more sedentary as the years go by. They lose lean body tissue and grow proportionately fatter, even on the same number of calories. This means that a sedentary woman of 50 who still looks slim and even weighs the same as she did when she was 20 may be made of as much as 50 percent fat or more! She may be eating very little to stay at that weight—and therefore becomes undernourished, encouraging further degeneration of lean tissues and bones, and making herself weak. But you *can* have firm, beautiful muscles at any age. Even after a lifetime of abuse and neglect, you have plenty of muscle to work with, which can be built up to quite impressive levels. The muscle cells aren't dead—they're just snoozing. Fat-burning activity preserves and builds lean muscle tissue, keeps the metabolic rate high, and helps prevent dramatic increases in body fat content while allowing you to eat well.

The pattern of your body fat distribution may change with age. For example, you may notice a thickening at your waist, while your buttocks and your face may hollow slightly owing to disappearance of subcutaneous fat there. This means that the Body Fat Ratio Scale may not give you as accurate an assessment of your body composition as it would a younger woman: you are also entitled to have a slightly higher level of body fat that is still considered "normal" for your age. If you get a reading on the Scale that seems much too high or far lower than you think is right, you may wish to use another simple method of determining your body fat content, which consists of a series of skin-thickness measurements taken with a special caliper. See p. 161 for buying information.

One of the most common afflictions of postmenopausal women is osteoporosis, which is marked by the increasing porosity, brittleness and thinning of bone. While some women may be more prone to develop osteoporosis than others, researchers now feel that the most prominent causes are poor calcium intake and a sedentary lifestyle. In order to remain strong, your skeleton *must* have bone-stressing activity. Cycling, rebound jogging and walking all provide the proper bone stimulation that can help you keep your skeleton intact. And the Better Body Shapers are excellent for maintaining the strength of bones in your arms, back and shoulders. As noted in Chapter 5, women over 35 should also be sure to get 1500 milligrams of calcium per day in their diets or with supplements.

You'll note that your Base Fat-Burning Heart Rate is much lower than that of a 30-year-old. But don't worry when you do your Sessions at that rate—you are getting the same workout a younger person does at her proper heart rate. A 45-year-old who exercises regularly will, in fact, be in much better shape than a 20-year-old who doesn't—and have a better figure.

If you have cardiovascular disease or high blood pressure, it may be caused or exacerbated at least in part by sedentary living. Regular fat-burning activity has been shown to reduce blood pressure and improve heart function in many people, and in some cases to eliminate the need for medication. Be sure to talk with your doctor, of course, before you start any exercise or diet program. And don't forget: you're entitled to a tax deduction if you have your doctor prescribe a stationary bike as part of the treatment for your condition.

8 / Questions and Answers

Q. Is cellulite different from other fat?

A. Most doctors claim that cellulite is simply fat that isn't being supported as well as it should be. Subcutaneous fat cells are held in a complex net of elastic collagen protein fibers. When these fibers are forced to support too much fat—or simply get too old—they may overstretch, stiffen and tear, pulling fat cells in various directions and creating the familiar "orange-peel" effect. Getting rid of as much fat as possible through fat-burning activity and diet, as well as shaping the muscles underneath the fat so they support it better, often eliminates the problem entirely. But according to Dr. Norman O. Orentreich, Associate Clinical Professor of Dermatology at the New York University School of Medicine, some women—particularly those who have taken oral contraceptives—have hardened patches of fat on thighs, hips and derrière which are stubbornly resistant even to proper diet and exercise. Dr. Orentreich and others have recently developed an office procedure, called suction curettage or lipectomy, which involves the surgical siphoning off of fat from these patches. Only small areas can be done at one time, at a cost of approximately $35 per visit. Dr. Orentreich advises that this still-experimental procedure should be done *only* after diet and exercise have first done all they can. A thigh with poor muscle tone will still look flabby, fat lumps or no fat lumps.

Q. I've gained ten pounds since I've been on the Pill. Can the Plan help me get rid of *them*?

A. Yes, unless you have special Pill-related metabolic problems. The hormones in oral contraceptives can cause water retention, but fat-burning activity often helps restore normal body water balance. You should, of course, restrict salt in your diet (and sugar, too, because it absorbs even more water than salt). The Pill can also cause more of the carbohydrates you eat to be stored as fat rather than be burned for energy, which makes you fatter *and* more tired. Again, fat-burning activity may be all you need to get your metabolism back to normal. But that may take some time. If you don't seem to be losing any weight, even after a few weeks on the Plan, you should see your doctor, and perhaps also consider the possibility of using another means of contraception.

Q. I have varicose veins. Will Fat-Burning Sessions make them worse?

A. No, it may help them a lot—and may prevent others from appearing. Your veins carry blood back to the heart, and the leg veins must work against gravity most of the time. A varicose vein happens when the valves inside the vein, which ordinarily snap shut to prevent the backward rush of blood, become weak and do not close all the way. This causes blood to pool in the vein, making it bulge. If your leg muscles are not in good shape, the problem is worsened, because leg muscles are the heart's auxiliary pumps, helping to return blood to the heart. When you do any fat-burning activity, you strengthen both these leg-muscle "pumps" and the muscularity of the vein walls. This can reduce varicose veins dramatically, and even help them disappear. Do check with your doctor, however, before starting any physical activity.

Q. What about the little tiny red veins on my thighs? Will exercise make them go away?

A. "Spider" veins often appear and disappear spontaneously, but fat-burning activity can help clear them up. The stubbornest ones can be destroyed with injections by a dermatologist.

Q. My waist is very small, but I've got really wide hips and big thighs. Will the Body Fat Ratio Scale still work on me?

A. The Body Fat Ratio Scale was developed from measurements of women of all shapes and sizes, so it should be accurate for most women. However, if you feel your figure has exceptionally unusual proportions, you can order a Slim Guide Skinfold Caliper from Creative Health Products, 50 Saddleridge Road, Plymouth, Michigan 48170 for $19.95 postpaid; call toll-free, 1 (800) 742-4478 (Michigan residents call 1 [313] 453-5309) to order on your credit card. It is a device used by physiologists and physicians that allows you to take subcutaneous-fat measurements easily at a few different places on your body. Like the Body Fat Ratio Scale, it tells you your body fat level and also helps you accurately monitor your fat loss on the Plan. The Slim Guide may also be used by women who weigh more than 171 pounds or are over 40, and by men.

Q. My parents were both overweight. Doesn't that mean that part of my problem is in my genes?

A. Overweight is a classic case of the cooperative effects of nature and nurture. At this point, scientists don't know how much heredity has to do with making people fat. A slower inborn metabolism and a slight tendency to make excess fat cells *may* predispose one to being chubbier than average. And fat persons may also be born with less of what is called "brown" fat than naturally thin people; brown fat tends to be much more metabolically active and apt to burn itself off at a higher rate than the more common "white" fat. But children in fat families are raised to eat the same way their parents do, and their activity level is almost always the same—meaning it is non-existent. Rather than accepting a fat fate, many offspring of fat parents are now slim—but only because they have made critical changes in eating and activity habits.

Q. I have lost and gained weight many times, and my breasts are really sagging. What do you think of plastic surgery?

A. First of all, you should do all the Breast Shapers for *at least* the six weeks you'll be on the Plan—and preferably for twelve weeks. Try to work up to 10-pound weights. This will let you see how your breasts look after they've gotten the maximum backup support from your pectoral muscles. Then, if the breast tissue itself still looks very saggy, you might consider having a relatively simple bit of plastic surgery called a breast lift. During this procedure, skin from beneath the breast is removed and the remaining skin is sewn together, which makes a much tighter, firmer "package" for the interior breast tissue. This means stretch marks are much less noticeable and may even be snipped away. Scarring is minimal or non-existent, since breasts heal well, and results are usually terrific. A breast lift costs anywhere from $2500 to $4500, but is fully tax-deductible. Contact your local medical society for referral to a board-certified plastic surgeon who is skilled in this type of breast surgery.

Q. I have always had terribly painful menstrual cramps, and I've heard that exercise helps. Will the Plan help me get rid of them?

A. No matter what your high school gym teacher told you, exercise doesn't do a thing for cramps. But there is at long last a class of drugs, formerly used for arthritic pain, that can forever end your agony. These non-narcotic pain-killers eliminate even the worst cramps by inhibiting the production of certain prostaglandins, which are hormonelike substances that cause uterine muscles to cramp. See your gynecologist for a checkup to make sure there's no other reason for your cramps, and if there isn't, ask for a prescription for one of these miracle drugs: Motrin, Ponstel or Anaprox.

Q. I get really bloated before my period. Can the Plan help?

A. Very likely. But first you need to understand the various causes of premenstrual water retention. Certain female hormones released in your system at that time attract water like magnets. If you take oral contraceptives, you get an extra dose of similar hormones. This water retention can be further aggravated by a deficiency of vitamin B_6 that often accompanies Pill use. You can take a supplement, if you wish, and see if that helps. High intakes of salt and sugar can cause the problem in a woman who would otherwise have no premenstrual bloating. Cutting down on salt and sugar is a good idea for everyone anyway, but is especially important before your period. Being sedentary messes up your body's water balance too, so fat-burning activity can solve the rest of the problem, as well as stimulate circulation so your ankles don't puff up. If your problem persists after following all this advice, *don't* take over-the-counter diuretics—see your doctor.

Q. I've heard that exercising can cause women to lose their periods. Can that happen to me on the Plan?

A. Women who regularly engage in truly strenuous activity—marathon runners, ballet dancers and gymnasts—sometimes experience amenorrhea, or loss of menstruation, due, in some cases, to *extremely* low levels of body fat. Rest assured, this is *not* going to happen to you on the Plan. In any case, this has never been shown to be a permanent condition, nor has it been shown to impair a woman's ability to have children once she has allowed her body fat percentage to rise again by cutting down slightly on exercise. But if ever you experience menstrual irregularities you haven't had before, you should of course see your gynecologist to find out what may be wrong.

Q. If I wear a sauna suit during my Fat-Burning Sessions, won't that make me lose fat even faster?

A. You should never wear rubber or plastic clothing during *any* kind of exercise. All it will do is make you lose water (which will be rapidly replaced) and minerals, whose absence will weaken you. It will also prevent the dissipation of heat that is generated by physical activity, which can send your body temperature dangerously high. Always wear light, comfortable, absorbent, loose-fitting clothing during physical activity.

Q. Can I follow the Plan at a health club?

A. You can if it has the right equipment. But be sure not to waste your money; a serious health club does not have any motorized machines that promise to do the work for you. (A motorized treadmill is an exception—you are still doing the walking or jogging.) You should look for good stationary bicycles, and a supply of dumbbells, and/or Nautilus or Universal weight-lifting machines (which you must be instructed to use properly). Don't use the sauna or steam room until you have cooled off sufficiently after your Fat-Burning Session. And make sure your club has a knowledgeable, nonpushy staff.

Q. Some beauty spas are advertising passive muscle-firming using electricity. Does it work?

A. It would seem that lying on a table snoozing while a machine zaps your flab away would be a blissfully lazy way to shape up. So naturally, I tried it. Electrodes were strapped to various parts of my naked body. The current was switched on, and a deep vibrating sensation could be felt within my stomach and thigh muscles, which soon began contracting in small rhythmic spasms. It was fairly pleasant until suddenly one of my buttocks began twitching so violently I nearly flipped off the table. The Food and Drug Administration would not have approved of the whole thing, since muscle-stimulation equipment, while authorized as effective for use in physical-therapy programs, has not officially been proved useful for weight loss or any other cosmetic purpose. A machine that pummels, vibrates or jiggles sundry parts of your anatomy can only throw your weight around, not off.

Q. Can massage help me lose fat?

A. Having a massage is one of the all-time great sensual experiences. It can definitely unkink tight muscles and improve circulation, and it feels great after exercise. *But it cannot break down fat.* No passive physical manipulation of any kind can get rid of fat, or make fat cells more eager to give up their contents. In fact, *too* vigorous manipulation of skin and underlying tissues can permanently damage the supportive collagen fibers that hold up fat cells, and thereby make flesh sag even more.

Q. I really like to dance. Can't I use dancing as a fat-burning activity?

A. Absolutely—just put on a favorite old or new record and boogie—or do the Charleston, the Lindy or the Twist. As long as your keep your legs moving continuously for 30 minutes, and check to see if you are at your Base Fat-Burning Rate, you'll get a very good, even a great workout. You may also count a vigorous night at the disco as a Fat-Burning Session. Or you may wish to join an aerobic dance class. But beware—these classes can be very discouraging to the beginning fat burner, because they are often led by young athletes or professional dancers who exhort you to keep up the pace at all costs. You must remember that all you *ever* need to do is keep going at your own pace. At first this may require nothing more vigorous than raising your heels barely off the floor in time to the music. But *you are getting the same workout* as the young contortionists next to you. My aerobic dance class was filled with college freshmen, some of them jazz and ballet dancers who could touch the ceiling with their toes. Compared with them, I was (and am) about as flexible as a stale pretzel. But I could outlast some of them, because I was and am in good *aerobic* shape. And we all had a great time.

Q. Why haven't you recommended swimming?

A. Swimming is indeed an excellent cardiovascular exercise and all-around muscle shaper. However, there are a couple of reasons why I didn't include it as a Plan alternative. First of all, it requires a pool, which you have to make a regular effort to get to. Second, your arms and your back are in worse initial aerobic fat-burning shape than even your legs at this point, and it would take a lot of dedication and effort to even get to a point where swimming would do you much good within six weeks. And swimming doesn't seem to pare off body fat quite as fast as other activities, even though it uses lots of calories. If you are still determined to swim, however, note that your correct Base Fat-Burning Heart Rate should be 13 beats per minute lower than usual, owing to the effects of reduced gravity. Do *continuous* laps using any stroke for 30 minutes. It doesn't matter how slowly you swim. You can even alternate using a kickboard with using your arms until they are stronger. Swimming is also quite good for very overweight people or those with painful joints, because it is not a weight-bearing exercise. It does *not* help prevent osteoporosis, however, for the same reason.

Q. How about jumping rope?

A. Jumping rope is terrific for fat loss and for firming lots of muscles. But in order to jump without having the rope go limp, you have to be coordinated, and not trip and fall down as I do. You also have to maintain a certain speed, which automatically elevates your heart rate way above your Base Fat-Burning Heart Rate. Jumping rope is, therefore, too strenuous for someone who is just starting a conditioning program.

Q. I was a real athlete in high school. Why am I so flabby now?

A. Because fitness didn't graduate with you. It doesn't matter if you were the biggest jock in the locker room—once you stop being athletic, you stop being fit. Muscles do not magically stay in shape for decades, but instead soon accommodate themselves to whatever level of activity is demanded of them. Within two weeks of stopping an aerobic fat-burning activity, you lose about a quarter of your fitness; within two months, you lose half. So unless you are currently doing something *regularly* to stay fit, you're in no better shape than the person who never exercised. You do have one advantage, however: you may find it easier to get into shape, since you know what to expect from each level of training and since you may still be a "natural athlete." But it's best to remember this motto: use it or lose it.

Q. I can see that my muscles need some firming, but I'm afraid of what will happen if I start doing the Better Body Shapers and then stop. Won't my muscles turn into fat?

A. Muscle and fat are two different types of cells, so one cannot possibly turn into the other. All that will happen if you stop exercising a particular muscle is that it will simply shrink back to the way it was before you started. If you then eat enough to gain weight, the fat cells over the muscle will, of course, obligingly fill up again. Then it's business as usual—flab. That's exactly what happens to body builders and football players who stop pumping iron and crushing their kneecaps.

Q. I'm a waitress and I'm on my feet all day. Don't I already get enough fat-burning activity that way?

A. The fact that you (and anyone who spends the day on her feet) do move around on the job gives you a health edge over people who are completely sedentary. Your heart is probably more fit. Your bones will certainly be stronger. But while you feel that your job keeps you in motion constantly, you are actually moving in a series of fits and starts, which prevents you from keeping your heart rate up high and long enough to improve your fitness. And if you are still overfat despite your job, it's obvious your exercise and dietary habits aren't what they should be. Once you start doing regular Fat-Burning Sessions, you'll soon find that your job will be much less tiring, because you will have begun to develop the reserve stamina you need. Since your poor feet need a rest, stationary cycling is probably the best activity for you.

Q. How can you say that protein diets don't work? My friends go on them all the time, and they always lose lots of weight really fast.

A. Protein diets are indeed the fastest way to lose *weight*— but not fat. When you eat a lot of protein and little or no carbohydrates, your body must use much of that protein for energy. Making lots of protein into glucose overworks your liver, and especially your kidneys, which must dilute and flush out the toxic by-products of protein and incomplete fat breakdown. (Fat can't be broken down cleanly without carbohydrates.) This requires water—plenty of water—which is leached from muscles and other body tissues. That's why protein dieters urinate a lot, and often feel tired and weak. But no matter how much water you drink, you can't keep up with the amount of water you need to process all that protein. Along with the water you lose with your glycogen, fluid loss adds up to a dramatic loss of pounds—at least in the first week. Still, you haven't lost any more fat than you would have on any other diet. Worse, you can even *gain* weight if you're eating too many calories—a gain that will be masked initially by the water weight loss but will show up as a cruel shock when you stop dieting and the water comes back. If the protein you're eating is mostly in the form of meat, you're getting an unhealthful dose of saturated fat. You're also weakening your bones, because excessive protein causes calcium to be lost in your urine. A final question for you: are all those friends *still* skinny after their last protein diet?

Q. Isn't fasting good for you once in a while? I've heard it cleans out the toxins in your system.

A. When you consume nothing but fruit juice or water, everything that happens on a low-calorie diet is simply stepped up to the maximum. Your body eats up its glycogen quite quickly, then goes to work on your muscles. Your brain begins to feed on emergency rations called ketones, the partially burned by-products of fat breakdown. Glucose shortage can also cause the euphoric lightheadedness easily confused with a religious experience, and too many ketones can cause the blood and tissues to become dangerously acidic. The only toxins in your body that need to be cleaned out are those produced by eating a diet too high in protein and/or fat and too low in fiber, or by fasting.

Q. What about an all-fruit diet?

A. Turning your intestines into a giant fruit cup does nothing but give you diarrhea—which, of course, makes you lose water weight. But this in turn can result in a loss of vital substances called electrolytes, which control nerve impulses and heart rhythm. Also, there is virtually no protein in such a diet, meaning your muscle tissue will get flushed down the toilet along with all that water. An all-fruit diet is just that—fruity.

Q. I'm really hooked on diet soda. Is it okay?

A. First of all, diet sodas contain artificial sweeteners, which, as I've noted, I prefer not to use regularly. But there are other reasons I can't feel comfortable recommending saccharin-containing diet sodas as part of a diet that is supposed to help make your body better. First of all, the saccharin currently used in many diet sodas is sodium saccharin. Sodium is salt, which you already get too much of in your diet and which makes you retain water. So drinking diet sodas all day can actually make you *heavier* and fatter-looking. Diet colas also contain phosphorus. While phosphorus is needed to combine with calcium and form bone tissue, too much phosphorus upsets the delicate proportion between the two and causes calcium to be excreted in the urine. Since calcium loss is already a major nutritional problem in women, it doesn't make sense to make things worse by drinking diet sodas all day. So you may drink diet sodas if you wish. But if you want a soft drink that badly, have a real one, with sugar, once in a while. Ginger ale is not that sugary or fattening. Better yet, get into the habit of drinking plain soda water with a slice of lemon, or mixed with fruit juice. And there's always plain water.

Q. I'm a caffeine addict. Is that bad?

A. It depends. Caffeine, which is found in coffee and regular and diet colas (and whose cousins theophylline and theobromine are found in tea and chocolate), is a powerful central-nervous-system stimulant. It does help wake you up, and it helps release sugar and fat into your bloodstream to be used for energy. But an excess of caffeine can also make you jumpy and tense, elevate your blood pressure and contribute to breast soreness before your period. So cutting down on your total caffeine intake is a good idea. Try to limit yourself to two cups of real coffee, tea or cola per day. Drink herbal teas, ginger ale and water instead.

Q. Does any diet drug work?

A. Pills containing phenylpropanolamine hydrochloride do dull your appetite, which of course gives you the temporary willpower you need to eat less. The Food and Drug Administration has approved pills containing the drug as safe and effective if used in the proper doses. However, a report summoned by the FDA from an independent panel noted that even the proper dosage can cause high blood pressure and heart-rhythm irregularities in susceptible individuals. (And even without the caffeine they so often contain, the pills can also make an ordinarily calm person like me nervous: I got so jittery on them the cheesecake kept falling off my fork.) Other diet preparations contain drugs that numb your tongue, so that that doughnut supposedly doesn't taste as good, or substances that swell in your stomach so that you supposedly feel full. None of these pills burns your fat off, of course; it's the diets they come with that cause weight loss to occur the usual dreary way. Nor do they teach you good permanent eating habits—so you don't stay slim for long. Prescription diet pills containing amphetamines, or "speed," which temporarily rev up the metabolism and decrease appetite, can cause severe depression, nervous-system damage and, if overused, heart failure. They are no longer prescribed solely for weight loss by responsible physicians.

The severely overweight individual, for whom ordinary diet and exercise alone is not speedy or effective enough, may soon find help from current weight-control research. Among the recent discoveries are the hormone cholecystokinin (CCK), which is produced in the intestines in normal persons in response to a meal and which acts as a powerful appetite suppressant in the brain; naloxone and naltrexone, which block the opiatelike effect food has on the brains of the obese, and the amino acid phenylalanine, which takes part in the production of the appetite-depressing neurotransmitter norepinephrine in the brain. There is also the old standby, thyroxine, administered to individuals who are short of this metabolism-stimulating thyroid hormone. None of these aids will take the place of proper diet and exercise; they are simply prospective aids to healthful fat reduction.

Q. What about starch blockers? They were the answer to my prayers. . . .

A. For a few seemingly idyllic months in 1981, the "miracle" pill that supposedly prevented starch from being digested and turned into fat was flying off drugstore shelves and being eagerly gobbled up along with mounds of macaroni. Even some government researchers confided to me that starch blockers looked promising, not necessarily for dieting—starch is an important nutrient—but perhaps for preventing the effects of an occasional spaghetti binge from appearing on one's hips the morning after. Despite unsubstantiated claims that the pills worked for some people, resulting in weight loss, they proved to cause bouts of gas and diarrhea in others, in some cases so severe as to require hospitalization. The Food and Drug Administration soon blocked sales, since the active ingredient in starch blockers and its various formulations had not been adequately tested for safety and was found by independent researchers to be ineffective. The whole concept of blocking starch is shaky anyway, since it is too much protein, fat and sugar in your regular diet that has made you fat, *not* too much starch.

Q. Is a vegetarian diet healthful?

A. Those who eat a *strictly* vegetation diet can be very well nourished if they take a supplement of vitamin B_{12}, which is found only in animal foods. A diet that is heavily vegetarian, containing small amounts of animal products, is consumed by the healthiest people in the world, meaning they have far lower incidences of heart and artery disease, diabetes and many types of cancer. It's a diet that isn't fattening; you can stuff yourself with broccoli and still not take in that many calories, since vegetables are bulky and contain little or no fat. You can easily convert your Better Body Diet to a part-time vegetarian diet simply by getting your protein more often from beans eaten with rice, corn or grains—which together make up the same high-quality "complete" protein found in animal products—and/or by combining starchy and other vegetables and grains with plenty of dairy products, or small amounts of meat, fish or poultry. Eating no red meat is a choice some people make to cut down on saturated fat, but it may also severely limit iron intake. For health and permanent svelteness, just add more vegetable entrées to your menus, and have a lot of "salad days." Vegetarian cooking *isn't* just soybeans and granola; it's pasta, eggplant Parmigiana and chili. Consult classic Italian, Spanish, Mexican and Indian cookbooks for old and new recipe ideas.

Q. Should I shop in health-food stores?

A. Yes and no. A health-food store is a good source of whole-grain breads, grains and beans—but your supermarket may carry these things, too. Beware overpriced "organic" vegetables and fruits, unless you know whose backyard they came from. A home-grown tomato certainly tastes better than those gassed pink golf balls in cellophane, and it may possibly contain more vitamins and minerals than one from a megafarm. You cannot, however, protect yourself against pesticides, because they permeate the soil virtually everywhere in the United States. Just be sure to wash your produce very well before eating.

Q. Margarine is better than butter, isn't it?

A. Not necessarily. Margarine has the same number of calories as butter, so it's not less fattening. One of the supposed health reasons to choose margarine is to cut down on artery-clogging saturated fats. However, for polyunsaturated fats to be hardened, they must be partially hydrogenated, or saturated, with hydrogen—producing substances called "trans fats," which some experts consider carcinogenic. If you do choose to use margarine, pick one that lists liquid corn or safflower oil as its main ingredient on the label. Avoid margarines that contain palm-kernel, cottonseed or coconut oil, since they may contain an even higher percentage of saturated fat than butter. And when you want butter, *eat* butter. It is total fat content in your diet that matters; a high combined intake of saturated and polyunsaturated fats is correlated with high rates of many types of cancer.

Q. Isn't honey or brown sugar better than white sugar?

A. No. The minuscule amounts of minerals do not compensate for the fact that honey is a pure dose of sugar. I use honey in my tea because it tastes good, not because it has any health virtues. Alert to the increasing diet and health consciousness of consumers, food manufacturers cleverly disguise sugar by calling it corn sweetener, corn syrup, beet sugar and various words ending in "ose." Some try to bamboozle you with such "natural"-sounding names as brown, turbinado or beet sugar. The most hilariously brazen of all is "natural refined sugar." Of course it's *natural*—it comes from sugar cane! But no matter what you call it, it's still sugar. And too much sugar, of course, makes you fat.

Q. Just what is cholesterol? Do I have to watch my intake of it on the Plan?

A. Cholesterol is a fatty alcohol which is found in high concentrations in and around your brain cells, and among other functions, is critical to the production of sex hormones. It is mainly manufactured in your body, but is also derived from animal products such as meat, organ meats, whole-milk dairy products, shellfish and egg yolks. An excess of serum (blood) cholesterol has been linked to heart and artery diseases. Ordinarily the body regulates its cholesterol production in response to dietary intake; however, in some individuals this feedback mechanism is defective, and they must watch their dietary intake of cholesterol. There is growing evidence that it isn't simply an abundance of cholesterol that boosts the body's cholesterol production or causes heart and artery diseases, but rather the total intake of fats as well as the relative proportions of certain cholesterol-depositing and cholesterol-removing substances in one's bloodstream. Fat-burning activity has been shown to increase the quantity of the cholesterol-removing substances and to lower blood fats. Since cholesterol- and fat-containing foods are frequently the same, it makes sense to limit the intake of such foods. The current recommended daily dietary intake of cholesterol is 300 milligrams per day or less; one egg yolk contains 240 milligrams.

But do bear in mind that a premenopausal female who does not smoke, exercises regularly, has healthy serum-cholesterol and blood-fat levels, is not on the Pill and is not overweight is at very low risk for getting heart disease. I fit all the above qualifications. So while I do watch my *total* fat intake, when a recipe calls for cream, or a warm slice of fresh bread cries out for butter, I use it. I also eat liver, shellfish and plenty of eggs—foods that are high in cholesterol but are low in total fat and extremely nourishing, because they are chock-full of protein, vitamins, trace minerals and other substances that are hard to come by in other foods. If for medical reasons you must monitor your intake of cholesterol, you may make a tasty omelet or scrambled eggs using only one egg yolk and three whites. Feed the extra yolks to your dog—they're good for her coat.

Q. Do I need to worry about food additives?

A. With the exception of the extra nitrates and nitrites used in meat, which seem to have a very strong cancer-causing potential (eliminated if the food also contains sodium ascorbate or ascorbic acid, both vitamin C), preservatives are not the dreaded poisons some people think they are. In fact, BHA and BHT may help prevent cancer and other types of cell damage that contribute to aging. Artificial flavorings, especially fruit flavors, aren't so bad either, because they are often the very same chemicals found in the actual fruits. What you should not be eating is artificial food *colorings*, unless they are "natural," such as annato and turmeric (spices) or beta carotene (a precursor of vitamin A). But you can eliminate much of the worry by remembering the premise of the Better Body Diet: you shouldn't be eating very many foods that have been tampered with in the first place. If a food needs that much sprucing up, it must have been dead a long time— or perhaps it never lived at all. And if you don't trust what you're reading on a food label, or feel you would need a Ph.D. in chemistry to decipher it, why on earth would you want to put it into your body?

Q. Are there any commercial cereals that fit the requirements of the diet?

A. Instant or regular Quaker Oats, Grape-Nuts, Shredded Wheat, Puffed Wheat, Puffed Rice, Maltex, Instant Ralston and most hot cereals are old standbys made from whole grains and unadulterated by too much added sugar or fat. When in doubt, read labels. Granola, by the way, a popular "health"-food item, is no nutritional bargain if it's made with coconut oil or other fats.

Q. I seem to be having trouble losing weight on 1200 calories a day. What should I do?

A. If you are under 5′2″, or have a very small frame or a particularly stubborn metabolism, you may need to use the Fat Loss Booster Diet for a few days each week to maintain your fat loss. This means no added fat or sugar. You must *not* skimp on the other nutrients!

Q. What do I do if I go off my diet?

A. So you go nuts and eat a pound of Godiva chocolates! *Don't* punish yourself or starve for the next two weeks— it's not such a big deal. You are not bucking for sainthood here. Just realize it will take you a little longer than planned to lose your 10 pounds. You can always compensate for the extra calories by going on the Fat Loss Booster Diet for a couple of days. Or you can add another Fat-Burning Session that week. But be sure to fully enjoy your binge!

Q. I have a problem I'm really ashamed of. I'm a compulsive eater, and I can't stick to a diet for long. Can the Plan cure me?

A. It's an essential part of your "cure." But first you must stop hating yourself. Compulsive eating is not a crime or a sign you are a greedy or bad person. It is an expression of perfectly human needs and fears you must begin to deal with in a healthier way. Right now, you are trying to fill a bottomless pit of emotional hunger inappropriately with food. There is plenty of professional help out there for people with eating disorders, in the form of group therapy and individual counseling. Don't be ashamed of seeking help—you are in as much pain as someone with a broken arm. You will also benefit from reading the superb analysis of compulsive eating and female fatness, *Fat Is a Feminist Issue* (Berkeley Books, 1981) by Susie Orbach. But you should also realize that the yo-yo dieting you've suffered through all these years has contributed greatly toward your problem. Dieting too severely and too often causes perfectly *normal*, outrageous hunger pangs that demand to be satisfied, and screws up your appetite controls—as has eating a lot of the surgary, starchy, fatty foods that are the binger's favorites. Also, you (along with the rest of the world) haven't been moving your body much. All this means your metabolism is messed up. So you need the same things everyone else reading this book does: fat-burning activity, and a sensible way of eating that helps you get slim while satisfying your appetite and your nutritional needs. While therapy can handle part of your problem, the Plan is here to take care of the rest, so you will at last have the better body you've always wanted *and* the ability to keep it.

Q. The only diet I seem to be able to follow is one that makes me eat precise quantities, and gives me menus to follow. Can you recommend a diet that will still give me the same results as the Better Body Diet?

A. You can take advantage of a unique computerized weight-reduction service called FITcomp, Inc., which can provide you with a fourteen-day diet composed of foods of your own choosing. For a questionnaire and full information, write to FITcomp, Inc., 512 Soule Blvd., Ann Arbor, Michigan 48103.

Q. Will the Plan do anything for my skin?

A. Several recent studies have shown that people who engage in regular, vigorous fat-burning activity have tighter, smoother, thicker and stronger skin and even fewer wrinkles than their sedentary contemporaries regardless of age! Fat-burning activity will also make you sweat a little, which can help clean out your pores. And it will give your skin a rosy glow throughout the day, due to increased blood circulation. All of these can make you look many years younger.

Q. How will the Plan affect my general health?

A. By improving your general fitness, the Plan will greatly improve your health. First of all, fat-burning activity will shape up your heart and your entire cardiovascular system. Along with strengthening muscles, Fat-Burning Sessions and Better Body Shapers stimulate growth of the connective tissues that support muscles and bones, which helps protect joints and bones from injury. They also strengthen bones themselves, which helps prevent osteoporosis, the bone-thinning disease that often occurs in postmenopausal women. Fat-burning activity can also play a role in preventing or controlling heart and artery disease, arthritis, high blood pressure, diabetes and, of course, obesity, which often sets the stage for the foregoing maladies. A fit body also recuperates from illness and surgery much faster. While being in good shape can't cure or prevent all diseases, it certainly does put the odds in your favor.

Q. I have always had trouble sleeping, and in the morning it shows. Is there any help for that?

A. I had always been a "light" sleeper myself. It took me forever to drift off, and if I awoke to, say, the distant crashing of moth wings, I could not get back to sleep. Once I became more active, I found I could sleep much more deeply and get more out of fewer hours. Physical activity acts as a natural sleeping pill, because it induces the right kind of physical sleepiness at the end of the day, and frees you of the restless mental fatigue that keeps you fitfully awake. Don't have a Fat-Burning Session immediately before going to bed, however—it might rev you up *too* much.

Q. I have diabetes. Can I go on the Plan?

A. You *must not* alter your prescribed diet or begin any type of physical activity without first consulting your physician. But depending on the type of diabetes you have, you may benefit greatly from following the Plan. Recent research has shown that regular fat-burning physical activity can help regulate blood sugar and decrease insulin needs in many diabetics. A high–complex-carbohydrate, low-fat diet (without sugar, of course) is the kind currently being recommended to control both juvenile-onset (Type I) and adult-onset (Type II) diabetes. Loss of weight, a correct diet and regular physical activity are often the only measures needed to control the latter type of diabetes—and all these elements are included in the Plan. If you have insulin-dependent diabetes, it is essential that you and your physician work closely to monitor any changes in insulin requirements necessitated by your increased physical activity and weight loss.

Q. Will smoking affect my progress on the Plan?

A. You will be able to lose weight on the Plan whether you smoke or not. But I can't honestly declare you will end up with a much better body. There's no need to discuss the multitude of compelling reasons why you shouldn't be smoking; you already know why—so I won't try to tell you to stop. But I do hope you try to smoke less while you're on the Plan, since smoking cuts way down on your wind, which in turn impairs your ability to bring in the oxygen you need to burn fat. There is some good news: many people find they have a reduced desire to smoke when they begin doing regular fat-burning activity. And once you quit, your body bounces back very quickly and your lungs even clean themselves out, no matter how long you've been smoking.

Q. What if I stop the Plan because I'm sick?

A. Stay in bed, relax and get well. You can continue to stay on the Better Body Diet, if you wish—you won't lose much lean tissue in a few days. Just start doing your Fat-Burning Sessions when you feel better. If you break an arm or leg, however, you should do your Better Body Shapers to prevent muscle degeneration.

Q. How can I stay on the Plan while I'm on vacation?

A. For most people—including me—a vacation is a time for uninhibited enjoyment of food. But between the croissants and the Sacher tortes you should at least try to keep moving. Walking is the best way to see the sights of any city. Doing so might prevent you from gaining weight—and you might even lose some. And you will, of course, still be steadily improving your fat-burning capacity, so that when you get home you need only start your diet again. Just be sure to pack comfortable shoes.

Q. My husband has seen the results of the Plan on me, and now he wants to go on it too. Will it work for him?

A. Absolutely. He follows the same fat-burning schedule as you do. As far as the Better Body Shapers are concerned, he can just think of them as weight lifting—because that's what they are: he just starts with 10- or 15-pound dumbbells for each exercise. To lose weight on the Better Body Diet, he can consume 1500–1800 calories, depending on his build, which means two more servings of meat, fish, or poultry and one or two more servings of starchy foods than are listed for you. He should lose at least 15 pounds in six weeks, simply because he's a man and therefore has a somewhat faster metabolism than you do, due to a larger muscle mass. If he wishes to measure and monitor his body fat level, he should get the Slim Guide Skinfold Caliper described on page 161.

9 | Maintaining Your Better Body the Lazy Way— Forever

Congratulations—you've done it! You've achieved the better body that was waiting inside you all this time!

First of all, you are 10 pounds lighter—maybe many more—than you were only six weeks ago. And for once in your life, those pounds you lost were 10 pounds of solid fat. If you want to know just how proud of yourself you ought to be, go to the supermarket and pick up 10 pounds of butter—or better yet, lard.

You have probably dropped at least a full size in pants and dresses, so you're going to have to get some new ones, which you richly deserve.

Your thighs haven't looked so firm in years. You can even wear shorts without feeling shy.

You can't believe it, but your breasts really *are* higher and rounder and more prominent.

Now that you have lost the flab on the backs of your arms, you can wear barer, sexier tops.

In short, you like what you see in the mirror. No, you *love* it! And you didn't have to struggle or starve to get that way. Best of all, you don't have to struggle or starve to *stay* that way.

A FIRM FOUNDATION FOREVER

The foundation of your permanently better body is and always will be a good level of aerobic fitness. This is what you achieved during your Fat-Burning Sessions. If you do nothing else physical for the rest of your life, *it's critical that you do some sort of fat-burning activity on a regular basis.* This will keep you burning calories, help you maintain your weight and your figure, keep your heart and your entire cardiovascular system as well as your bones and joints strong and give you a limitless supply of energy.

You'll be pleased to know that maintaining your new improved metabolism and enhanced fat-burning power forever is even easier than achieving it. All you need to do is continue to do some kind of fat-burning activity at your Base Fat-Burning Rate for a minimum of three times a week. If you want to improve your fat-burning potential even more, you can increase the duration of your Sessions from 30 to 45 minutes or an hour, increase the frequency to five times a week or increase the intensity of your Session, working at a higher heart rate within your fat-burning range. Doing any one or all of these will greatly increase your caloric expenditure, so you can eat pretty much as you like.

To maintain the new firmness of your body parts, you simply continue to do any or all of the Better Body Shapers, using the weight for the number of sets and reps you had worked up to by week six. If you wish to continue building and shaping any part of you, just do your Shapers more often, and increase the weight you're using.

THE SPORT WITHIN

Even though you may have started out as a lazy person and still (and forever will) think of yourself as such, you have become pretty active over the last six weeks. While you were busy burning off fat and shaping various body parts purely for cosmetic reasons, you were simultaneously undergoing the kind of general conditioning an athlete goes through to prepare her body to engage in a sport.

You have more endurance and stamina, the attributes of the marathon runner. If you've done most of the Better Body Shapers, you have developed strength and flexibility you never had before. You have, in fact, become something of an athlete yourself!

While you may never wish to run in races or compete in arm-wrestling matches, you now have a general foundation of fitness that allows you to engage in one or any number of leisure-time activities you have always wanted to try.

Your first choice *must* always be some kind of aerobic, fat-burning activity. You already know the details about stationary cycling, rebound jogging and walking. You can continue to do these, of course. You can start an entirely new activity. Or you can mix any number of activities. Do whatever keeps you interested and happy.

Here's a rundown of fat-burning activities and sports you might want to consider doing seasonally, occasionally or from now on:

Jogging/Running

Yes, you may want to try jogging or running. (What's the difference? Some say running is anything faster than a 9-minute mile. Actually, running is whatever feels fast to *you*.) You need never go faster than a 12-minute mile to get all the fat-burning benefits. You don't even have to take your pulse, because carrying your own body weight automatically elevates your heart rate. Start by interspersing brisk walking with a minute or two of very slow jogging for a week or two. Keep shortening the interval until you can jog for 20–30 minutes, three or four times a week. I actually got involved so much in running at one point that I entered the L'eggs Mini Marathon, a 6.2-mile race, in New York's Central Park. It was a lot of fun jogging along in the park chatting with all the other first-timers (including one woman who was six months pregnant and another aged 61). I may never compete again, but I will always cherish the medal I got for finishing that one race.

Aerobic Dancing

You don't have to be graceful or even very flexible to enjoy this and get all its fat-burning benefits. There are plenty of aerobic dance records to which you can dance at home. If you join a class, it gives you a chance to be with people. Some instructors are a bit overenthusiastic and urge you to go all out, which isn't necessary. Nor must you kick your heels as high as the rubbery young creature next to you. To stay fit, you need only keep your heart at your correct Fat-Burning Rate. (Once in a while, when you are feeling particularly peppy, you may want to work very hard.) Wear running shoes, not ballet slippers, because you will do a lot of hopping. Whatever you do, have a good time. Disco dancing is also a great fat burner, as is tap dancing.

Bicycling

Biking outdoors is great exercise, and a great way to see the sights. But, as is not the case with indoor cycling, you may be interrupted by traffic, especially in the city. To get a continuous workout, you must pedal at least 8 miles in 40 minutes. Obviously, going up hills adds to the effort—but coasting down doesn't count.

Backpacking, Hiking

Just plain walking with a full backpack gives you a terrific workout. You can even plan backpacking/hiking vacations during which you can eat heartily and not gain an ounce.

Cross-Country Skiing

This is one of the most strenuous sports, even more so than long-distance running, because the arms are involved as well as the legs. But you don't have to do it for speed, just for fun. To some, an afternoon of slogging through the snowy countryside in woolly knickers is bliss.

Swimming

Swimming is wonderfully relaxing, and an excellent all-over body conditioner, even though it doesn't keep body fat level down as efficiently as other activities. However, though your heart and legs are presently in pretty good shape, you may find that swimming tires you very easily at first. While running, dancing and biking all rely on the leg muscles and are therefore somewhat interchangeable, swimming relies heavily on your shoulders, your arms and the big muscles in your back, all of which must be conditioned for aerobic work. This takes time, and the only way to do it is to keep swimming, slowly and regularly. A good way to train is to alternate using your arms with using a kickboard, so that you get a continuous workout while giving your arms a periodic rest. Note: Your correct Base Fat-Burning Rate while swimming will be 13 beats per minute lower than during the equivalent workout on dry land, owing to the absence of the extra work imposed by gravity.

OTHER ALTERNATIVES

If you aren't afraid of falling down a lot, you can try ice and roller skating.

Other sports, such as downhill skiing, horseback riding and tennis, can be aerobic if you can keep them up long and skillfully enough. But you shouldn't rely on them for your main aerobic sessions. Just do them for fun, as you would golf, bowling, Ping-Pong, baseball, softball, volleyball, badminton, archery, knitting and sex.

Now that your muscles are reasonably strong, you might want to try yoga. Yoga will relax you, improve your flexibility and unkink parts of your body that get kinked during a deskbound day. Or you may want to take up ballet, modern dance, calisthenics or even karate.

The point is, of course, to *stay physical*. Having a body you feel more comfortable in, a body that you know you can trust to keep you moving for a reasonable amount of time and with a respectable amount of grace, opens up exciting new opportunities for you. You will inevitably have new physical—and mental—confidence in yourself. You may feel a new sense of adventure. Who knows?—you may even want to try your hand at skydiving, mountain climbing or white-water rafting. Okay, you're not, and never will be, *that* adventurous—but you can still enjoy the smug feeling that you *could* do them if you really wanted to, because now you've got what it takes!

IF YOU STOP . . .

Your body is very forgiving and adaptable. So if you stop exercising for a while, don't despair—it's *never* too late to start again. If you don't do anything for a week or two, you can usually resume your activity at the same level you had previously reached. If you drop off for a month, start at whatever level is comfortable. Your body doesn't fall to ruin in that amount of time, but it does need to be "reprimed." Do try, however, not to rest on your laurels for too long—or all you'll end up with is fat laurels.

FOR THOSE WHO NEED MORE TIME

Perhaps you have 10, 20, perhaps even 50 pounds or more to lose. You still have great reason to be proud of how far you've come, because by now you've probably lost at least 15 pounds. And you've begun making those all-important metabolic changes that will promote further fat loss and eventually keep you slim forever.

The *only* way to take off fat successfully is to give yourself enough time, and have enough patience. You have been bruised so much in the past by diets that didn't, *couldn't* work for you that you must give yourself a chance to get used to doing things right. It's time you stopped blaming yourself. Being overweight is not a crime; it's a disorder for which you needed sensible nutritional and physical guidance. Finally you've got it. So start feeling good about yourself and your body!

Whether you still have a little or a lot of fat to lose after six weeks, you can simply continue to follow the Plan as is. If you can increase the duration or the frequency of your Fat-Burning Sessions, you will lose fat faster.

It is perfectly safe to continue using the Better Body Diet for as long as you need to. But you don't have to stay on it all the time. You can take breaks, and instead eat the minimum number of calories it would take to maintain your target weight, which you figure by multiplying your goal weight by

12. As long as you continue to do your Fat-Burning Sessions, you will continue to lose fat, but at a slower pace.

The fads will come and go, but the physiological realities of weight reduction won't. If you have a setback, don't despair. You're human. We all are. You can always start again, and the Plan is always waiting here to help you. And in a few months, or a year from now, when you reach the weight you want to reach and discover your better body within, you'll *know* it was worth the wait!

YOUR PERSONAL MAINTENANCE CALORIE QUOTA

You have lost weight successfully on 1200 calories. To maintain your weight, you need to take in the number of calories that will supply you with the required amounts of all nutrients while also providing for your energy expenditure.

A *sedentary* woman who is at her correct weight needs approximately 12 calories per pound of body weight per day to maintain that weight. Because you are no longer sedentary, you are entitled to approximately 16 calories a day per pound of your new weight. So if the new lean you weighs 128, you should need at least 2048 calories per day to stay there.

That figure is, of course, an estimate. Every body is different, and you may require more or slightly fewer calories to maintain your weight. But you can start with this figure and see whether or not your weight fluctuates within a two-week period.

FEEDING YOUR BODY RIGHT FOR LIFE

Now that you've gotten down to your new weight, you may be tempted to toss the book aside and head for the kitchen. You've gotten rid of all those pounds. It's time to celebrate!

Yes, you should celebrate. But you must resist the temptation to add the additional calories you're going to be consuming to maintain your new weight all in one day. Even though you have been dieting sensibly, your body still viewed it as a reduction. If you bombard it with a large caloric intake all at once, too many of those calories will be converted into body fat. Instead, you should gradually add 100 or so calories to your diet every few days, and keep monitoring your weight.

You may see a pound or two come back for good—but don't worry, it's only water. Remember, you *can't* gain a pound of fat in a day unless you eat 3500 calories over your required caloric intake! Just don't encourage further water weight gain by eating anything excessively salty or sugary right away.

Beyond that, you must get one other simple fact straight: if you choose to go back to subsisting primarily on a diet of fatty, sugary junk food, you will have a junk body. The information provided in Chapter 5 wasn't just for six weeks—it's for *forever*. You are literally what you eat. To stay lean, you must eat lean. If you eat a lot of fat, a lot of you will be made of fat.

The average daily Western menu is currently composed, in terms of calories, of approximately 20 percent protein (mostly from fatty beef and dairy products), 40 percent fat (most of it saturated) and 40 percent carbohydrates (mostly in the form of sugar and refined-flour products). It is low in fiber, and deficient in some vitamins and minerals. In addition to making you fat, eating this way presents other definite health hazards. The high saturated-fat content of the diet increases your risk of heart and artery disease, while the high *total* fat content has proved to be a major causative factor in nearly all types of cancers, and specifically those of the breast and colon.

The following guidelines for a healthier and less fattening breakdown of nutrients by calories emerged from discussions with a number of nutritionists and from current nutritional research:

Protein

At least 12 percent, but not more than 20 percent, of calories. While you do need a certain amount of protein, you should not eat excessive amounts, because too much protein has been shown to interfere with calcium absorption and thus to cause bone deterioration. Instead of relying so much on meat, which comes along with fat, get more of your protein from other food sources, such as starchy vegetables, beans, grains and low-fat dairy products.

Carbohydrates

At least 50 percent of calories. Carbohydrates, in the form of starches, vegetables and fruits, should be the main source of your daily calories, and of those calories you will be adding to maintain your new weight. You should always get half or more of your bread and cereals and other grains and starchy vegetables in whole-grain or whole-food forms such as oatmeal, corn, whole-wheat bread, etc. But you may also eat some starch in the form of cakes, pastries and cookies, as long as they come within your maintenance calorie quota for the day and they are not regularly substituted for other nutrients. You should continue to eat plenty of fresh vegetables, including a green or yellow vegetable at *least* every other day—preferably every day—for vitamins C and A, and plenty of fruit, including a citrus or other vitamin C–containing fruit every day. Less than 10 percent of your daily calories should come from simple refined sugars, such as refined white sugar, brown sugar, honey and syrups.

Fats

No more than 30 percent of calories. This is the most negotiable element in your permanent weight-maintenance program. Dieting or not, you still don't need more than the same old 100–200 calories of fat to live on. So the amount of fat you eat is up to you. At a maintenance caloric intake of about 2000, a 30-percent fat inake is 600 calories of fat per day. That includes about 200 calories of fat found naturally in your food, plus 400 calories of fat you may consume in the form of butter, oil or other high-fat sources. Some experts I spoke with admitted privately that they felt 30 percent was still a high figure; populations with the lowest rates of cancer, heart disease and obesity consume only about 15 percent of their total daily calories in fat. But tastes are hard to change; we are very fond of fat. Just do try to keep your average fat intake over a week's time below the 30-percent level. Try to have fat-free days. Avoid large amounts of saturated animal fat (from fatty meats, whole-milk dairy products); artificially hydrogenated fats (found in margarine; look for those which contain liquid corn or safflower oil as the first ingredient) and coconut oil. At least two-thirds of the fats you do consume should be in the form of polyunsaturated vegetable oils if you are concerned about heart disease.

The specific amounts of food you will need to maintain your weight depend, of course, on your calculated personal maintenance calorie quota, which for most women will probably be between 1600 and 2000 calories per day. The following menu, based on the above guidelines, provides 1600 calories per day—the *absolute minimum* even the smallest woman must consume to fill her most basic nutritional requirements. It should be considered the *permanent foundation of your daily menu*, regardless of the additional calories to which you are entitled for weight maintenance. "Servings" are as defined in Chapter 5.

1600-CALORIE FOUNDATION DIET

7 servings starchy foods (including at least 3 whole-grain products and at least 1 starchy vegetable)

6 servings protein sources (lean meat, poultry, fish, organ meats, beans)

2 vegetables (including at least one green or yellow each day or every other day)

3 fruits (at least one citrus or other vitamin C–containing fruit per day)

2 servings of a dairy product (low-fat or skim milk, yogurt, cheese)

8 teaspoons fat (optional)

7 teaspoons sugar (optional)

To reach a maintenance caloric intake beween 1600 and 2000 calories, you should *not* add more servings of protein sources. Your extra calories should come primarily from carbohydrates, in the form of 1–3 more servings of starch (which supplies energy and some extra fat-free protein), at least 1–2 more servings of vegetables and 1–2 more servings of fruit. You may also add another serving of a dairy product. Use the food lists in Chapter 5 to guide you in assembling your maintenance menu.

After accounting for the calories in these foods, you may have room for a bit more fat. If you can stick to 8 teaspoons of added fat (or high-fat food) suggested on the Foundation

Diet, that's great, because the less fat you eat the better. Remember that you must keep in mind the fat naturally found in foods when accounting for daily fat intake.

You can have a little more sugar, too, if your calorie quota allows; in fact, you're better off eating a little more sugar than you are more fat. Alcohol should be considered a sugar substitute: 1½ ounces of hard liquor or 3½ ounces of wine is equivalent to 6 teaspoons of sugar.

HOW TO HAVE YOUR CAKE ... AND STAY SVELTE TOO!

Rather than cramping your eating style, these nutritional guidelines give you tremendous freedom while ensuring that you are nourishing your body. They even allow room in your menu for spareribs, ice cream, French fries, chocolate cake and all the other things that make life worth living. You can, in fact, eat anything and everything you want almost every day of your life while staying slim, just by following these guidelines for better eating forever:

Always Operate from a "Nutrient Base"

Your first responsibility to your body must be to feed it at least the minimum servings of food specified on the Foundation Diet. Once you accept that as an absolute, you won't have to worry about whether or not you are adequately nourished. You will also learn to think before you bite. Before you put a cake doughnut into your mouth, you might ask yourself, "Have I had enough whole-wheat or other whole-grain food or unrefined starches yet today?" Now that you know what your body must have to stay healthy, you will be less willing to put garbage into your mouth. And you won't hate yourself in the morning.

Juggle Those Carbohydrates

As you recall, you should get your starch (or a minimum of four servings on the Foundation Diet) from healthful sources such as whole-wheat bread, cereals, potatoes, corn, beans, etc. (These foods also contain the Fat Sponges and B vitamins you need to stay slim, so you should *want* to eat them.) But beyond those four servings (and occasionally, instead of them), you can apportion your calories in many delicious ways. For example, if you will be maintaining your weight at 2000 calories, you have 8 servings or, at 70 calories per serving, 560 calories of starch to play with. If you wish, you can spend 3–4 servings on a big piece of chocolate cake or a pile of cookies. Of course, there's sugar in the cake and cookies too, so you set aside some of your sugar calories. But sugar and starch are both carbohydrates, so they may be considered interchangeable. You may *not*, however, borrow calories from fruits, vegetables, dairy products or protein so that you can spend the day locked in a bakery. That risks your *health*, not to mention your waistline. And obviously the number of starch and sugar calories consumed must not exceed what you can afford to eat to maintain your weight.

Ration Fat

Let's face it: the tastiest things on earth are composed of not only starch and sugar, but also fat. So to have that piece of chocolate cake, you must set aside most or all of your fat calories too. To earn ice cream, you would set aside servings of a dairy product, sugar (or starch) *and* fat. Figuring out precisely how much fat is in a pastry or a rich sauce is an impossible task, however. If you want a fatty treat in any one day, you must resolve to ration your fat specifically for that one food, and use it nowhere else in your menu that day. If you decide to have ice cream at lunch, then you don't use any butter on your potato and you drink only skim milk at dinner. It's that simple. But it *works*.

Shift Proportions

You are no doubt currently accustomed to making a meal revolve around a meat entrée. It's time you learned that this is a fattening way to eat. But you don't have to become a vegetarian: instead of having a huge steak and a small potato and an even smaller green salad, have a small steak, two big potatoes and a *huge* salad. Make a habit of reaching for seconds and thirds of vegetables before having another slab of beef. If you make tasty fresh vegetable casseroles instead of the limp, overcooked mush that comes from a can, your family will come around to better eating, too.

Choose Nutrient-Dense Foods Most Often

If you choose most of your foods from those which offer the most nutrients for the fewest calories, you have even more room for treats, because you will save on total calories. Foods that work "nutritional overtime" in this fashion are salmon and sardines (protein and calcium), chicken and fish (protein, vitamins, minerals and little fat), dark leafy or other dark green vegetables (vitamins A and C, calcium, B vitamins, iron and other minerals), skim-milk dairy products (protein, calcium), beans (starch, protein, B vitamins, iron, fiber) and *all* whole-grain products (starch, protein, B vitamins, iron and fiber). Fill up your menu regularly with these nutritious "wonder" foods, and you'll always have lots of calories left for goodies after meeting those critical nutritional requirements.

. . .

These are all good rules to follow when planning your daily menu. But while it's important to keep track of what you eat in a day, it's more convenient and efficient to think in terms of what you consume in a week—especially in the case of fat. This allows you to have the inevitable high-fat, high-calorie "crazy" day without getting hysterical about gaining weight.

Say one day you have a breakfast of two croissants, a Big Mac for lunch and a huge platter of barbecued ribs for dinner. You have consumed about 50 percent of your calories that day in the form of fat, gone over your weight-maintenance calorie quota *and* shortchanged yourself on nutrition. The next two or three days, you simply eat very little or no fat, and lots of the nutrient-dense foods mentioned above. You can also cut calories to the Foundation Diet minimum of 1600, or to 1200, per day. By the end of the week, your fat intake will have averaged out to the desired 30 percent of calories, you haven't died of malnutrition—and you won't have gained an ounce! You can look back over your indulgences with nothing but fond memories. In time you will learn when you can afford to reach for something utterly without redeeming nutritional value, and when to reach for the salad. And you will be able to look in the mirror and smile!

So eat well, but wisely. If you don't know how to cook, learn. Expand your taste horizons. Eat more pasta. Sample new ethnic dishes. The world is a smorgasbord of great cuisines. *Mangia!*

WHAT IF ...

Like death and taxes, this is something you don't want to think about right now.

But let's get it over with. What if you forget yourself and . . . gain weight again?

If it doesn't happen, you're in the minority. (In fact, you're a little *scary*.) If you're a food lover, as I am, or merely human, you will at some point succumb to temptation. You may simply be resigned to gaining a few pounds every Christmas.

Believe it or not, you're in a much better position to *gain* weight than you have ever been before!

When you have a body that has become active and undergone the profound physical and chemical changes yours has, gaining a few pounds of fat is really not such a big deal. You have a whole new framework of shapely, firm muscles on your body—so a few extra pounds simply won't look the same as they did before. You can afford to carry more fat without *looking* fat.

Assuming that enough important nutrients (meaning a balance of protein and carbohydrates) are included along with your extra calories, you won't lose your lean tissue, even if you stop exercising at the same time. A brief bout of overeating *can't* make your body revert to its former fat-storing ways. The best possible course, however, is simply to do some kind of fat-burning activity through a holiday season or a vacation. That way, even if you *do* overeat enough to gain weight, you won't gain nearly as much as you would have if you'd ceased all extra physical activity at the same time. And you will drop the extra weight much faster, because you have maintained your metabolism at its usual snappy pace.

You don't even have to diet the extra pounds off if you don't want to. Just return to the number of calories that maintains your ideal weight, and your Fat-Burning Sessions will do the work for you. That is the healthiest way of all to lose fat. (If you ever do need to really *diet*, just go back to 1200 calories a day for a while.) And use your Body Fat Ratio.

Scale periodically, to make sure things aren't getting out of hand.

The best comfort of all is that it will simply be *harder* than ever before for you to gain fat weight—even if you *stuff* yourself for a day or two. You are simply burning off calories faster than you used to. Your leaner body is made of more muscle, which consumes more calories than your fatter body used to. And your appetite may be easier to control. You simply may not want to pack away the quantity of random scraps you used to before you knew what effect they would have. You and your body are now in better control of themselves than ever before.

SOUND BODY, SOUND MIND

The acquisition of your better body may start a chain reaction that can improve virtually all areas of your life—not the least of which is your *sex* life. You look better than ever. So naturally you'll feel more comfortable meeting new people—and they'll be more eager to meet you. Becoming physically active can make you more aware of your physical self, which can in turn help you recognize yourself as more of a sexual being. The new energy you have is absolutely sure to bring new zest to your relationships. Both outdoor and indoor sports will become *much* more fun!

A new body can lead to new confidence—and even give you a whole new outlook on life. Now that you're happier with your appearance, you won't want to hide in the shadows. And the fact that you have achieved one major goal—a better body—means you can achieve others. This can inspire you to get a new job, start a new career or even find a new lover. You feel you can meet any challenge—and you will.

As the ancient Greeks knew, a sound mind is truly inseparable from a sound body. To remain alert and active, your brain must get a regular supply of oxygen and nutrients, which is best supplied by a healthy heart and circulatory system. A fit body regularly produces a supply of chemicals far more potent than tranquilizers which help keep you more relaxed and cheerful, so daily problems that used to seem so bad don't bother you as much anymore.

In short, you are better for *life*.

And now I shall retire my better body to my couch, where I shall nibble on a bonbon or two, and raise a champagne toast to you and *your* better body.

Acknowledgments

I wish to express my appreciation to a number of people who provided the scientific foundations for the concepts in the book, as well as to those whose professional and personal support greatly smoothed the way toward its completion.

I thank William C. McArdle, Ph.D., Professor of Health and Physical Education at Queens College of The City University of New York and noted exercise physiologist, for his guidance and for graciously allowing me access to the research facilities at the college. I thank Victor L. Katch, Professor of Physical Education and Associate Professor of Pediatric Cardiology, School of Medicine, University of Michigan, and Frank I. Katch, Professor and Chairman of the Department of Exercise Science at the University of Massachusetts, for permission to include their Body Fat Ratio Chart in the text. I also thank Norman Orentreich, M.D., Clinical Associate Professor of Dermatology, New York University Medical Center, and Director of the Orentreich Medical Group, and Jerome Zuckerman, Ph.D., Director of the Cardio-Fitness Centers of New York, for their comments.

I would also like to express my gratitude to the experts in the field of nutrition who provided information both by phone and in scientific papers: among them Francis J. Cronin, Ph.D., Nutritionist, Nutrition Guidance and Education Research Division, Human Nutrition Information Service, U.S. Department of Agriculture, whose extensive guidance was especially appreciated; June L. Kelsay, Ph.D., Research Nutritionist, Human Nutrition Center, U.S. Department of Agriculture; Louis V. Alvioli, M.D., Shoenberg Professor of Medicine, Washington University School of Medicine, and Chairman of the Division of Bone and Mineral Metabolism, Jewish Hospital of St. Louis, and Jane Folkman, M.S., R.D., Nutrition Counselor, Joslin Diabetes Center, Boston.

I thank those few friends who have patiently tolerated my zeal-of-the-converted ravings about health and fitness and still remained friends, especially Ruth Gruen, who had a better body to begin with and will continue to have one forever if she only follows my advice.

I thank my sister, Robin Reedy, who lent not only her typing skills but her expertise as a veteran dieter to the preparation of the manuscript.

Thanks also to my literary agent, Beth Backman, for her efforts in getting my book into the right hands.

Finally, I thank those right hands, Joni Evans and Marjorie Williams, my splendid and skillful editors at Linden Press, who made the inevitable trimming of the fat from the early drafts a remarkably painless experience.

References

BOOKS

Bailey, C. 1978. *Fit or Fat?* Boston: Houghton Mifflin.

Bennett, W., & Gurin, J. 1982. *The Dieter's Dilemma: Eating Less and Weighing More.* New York: Basic Books.

Brody, J. 1981. *Jane Brody's Nutrition Book.* New York: W. W. Norton.

Carnes, V. & R. 1978. *Bodysculpture: Weight Training for Women.* New York: St. Martin's Press.

Cooper, M. & K. H. 1972. *Aerobics for Women.* New York: Bantam Books.

Fredericks, C. 1982. *Carlton Fredericks' Nutrition Guide for the Prevention & Cure of Common Ailments & Diseases.* New York: Simon and Schuster.

Katahn, M. 1982. *The 200 Calorie Solution: How to Burn an Extra 200 Calories a Day and Stop Dieting.* New York: W. W. Norton.

Katch, F. J., & McArdle, W. D. 1977. *Nutrition, Weight Control, and Exercise.* Boston: Houghton Mifflin.

Kunin, R. A. 1980. *Mega-Nutrition.* New York: McGraw-Hill Book Company.

Lyon, L., & Hall, D. K. 1981. *Lisa Lyon's Body Magic.* New York: Bantam Books.

McArdle, W. D.; Katch, F. I., & Katch, V. L. 1981. *Exercise Physiology.* Philadelphia: Lea & Febiger.

Pearson, D., & Shaw, S. 1981. *Life Extension: A Practical Scientific Approach.* New York: Warner Books.

Schwarzenegger, A., & Hall, D. K. 1979. *Arnold's Bodyshaping for Women.* New York: Simon and Schuster.

Watt, B. K., *et al.* 1975. *Handbook of the Nutritional Contents of Foods,* prepared for the United States Department of Agriculture. New York: Dover Publications.

Wurtman, J. J. 1979. *Eating Your Way Through Life: A No-Nonsense Guide to Good Nutrition for All Ages and All Eating Styles.* New York: Raven Press.

PERIODICALS AND NEWSLETTERS

Bennett, William. 1981. "The Tragedy of Anorexia Nervosa." *The Harvard Medical School Health Letter,* Department of Continuing Education, Harvard Medical School, Vol. VII, No. 2.

Editorial Staff. 1980. "Weight Control." *Ibid.,* Vol. VI, No. 2.

————. 1981. "An Update on the Cancer-Cholesterol Connection." *Ibid.,* Vol. VI, No. 12.

————. 1981. "HCG (Simeons) Diet Programs." *Ibid.*

————. 1981. "Osteoporosis—a Silent Epidemic." *Ibid.,* Vol. VII, No. 1.

————. 1981. "Low-Tar, Low-Nicotine—Are They Safer?" *Ibid.*

————. 1982. "An Update on Exercise—in Monkeys." *Ibid.,* Vol. VII, No. 5.

————. 1982. "The War on Cancer—Where Do We Stand?" *Ibid.,* Vol. VII, No. 6.

————. 1982. Is There Life After Jogging? *Ibid.*

Editorial Staff. 1982. "Exercise Bikes." *Consumer Reports,* Jan. 1982, pp. 38–40.

————. 1982. "Breads." *Ibid.,* Sept. 1982, pp. 438–43.

Editorial Staff. 1981. "Pregnant Jogger: What a Record!" *J. Amer. Med. Assn.,* Vol. 246, No. 3, p. 201.

————. 1981. "Seniors Needn't Go All Out for Fitness." *Ibid.,* p. 202.

Rozovski, S. J. 1982. "The Dietary Recommendations: What They Are and What They Mean." *Nutrition and Health,* Institute of Human Nutrition, Columbia University College of Physicians and Surgeons, Vol. 4, No. 1.

Winick, M. 1982. "Nutrition in American Women." *Ibid.*, Vol. 4, No. 1.

———. 1982. "Nutrition and Diabetes." *Ibid.*, Vol. 4, No. 4.

PUBLICATIONS

Editorial Staff. 1982. *Diet, Nutrition, and Cancer.* Committee on Diet, Nutrition, and Cancer. Assembly of Life Sciences, National Research Council. National Academy Press: Washington, D.C.

Federal Register. 1982. *Weight Control Drug Products for Over the Counter Human Use.* Department of Health and Human Services, Food and Drug Administration, Feb. 26, 1982, Vol. 47, No. 39.

PAPERS AND MONOGRAPHS

Alvioli, L. V. 1980. "Postmenopausal Osteoporosis." Symposium on Nutrition and Aging Bone Loss, Proceedings of the Federation of American Societies for Experimental Biology, pp. 2418–22.

Arky, R.; Wylie-Rosett, J., & El-Beheri, B. 1981. "Examination of Current Dietary Recommendations for Individuals with Diabetes Mellitus." *Diabetes Care*, Vol. 5, No. 1, pp. 59–63.

Epstein, L., & Wing, R. 1980. "Aerobic Exercise and Weight." *Addictive Behaviors* 5: 371–88.

Kelsay, J. L.; Behall, K. M., & Prather, E. S. 1978. "Effect of Fiber from Fruits and Vegetables on Metabolic Responses of Human Subjects." *Am. J. Clin. Nutr.*, 31:1149–53.

Lewis, D.; Katan, M.; Merkx, I., *et al.* 1981. "Towards an Improved Lipid-Lowering Diet." *The Lancet*, December 12, 1981, pp. 1310–13.

Light, L., & Cronin, F. J. 1981. "Food Guidance Revisited." *J. Nutr. Ed.*, Vol. 13, No. 2, pp. 57–62.

Linkswiler, H. M.; Zemel, M. B.; Hegsted, M., & Schuette, S. 1980. "Protein-Induced Hypercalciuria." Symposium on Nutrition and Aging Bone Loss, Proceedings of the Federation of American Societies for Experimental Biology, pp. 2429–33.

ABOUT THE AUTHOR

After deciding not to risk starvation as a singer and actress, Randi Blaun spent several years as an advertising copywriter and executive, and also wrote for television. She has written articles on a variety of topics, including food, dieting, exercise, health and fitness, as well as humorous pieces, for such publications as *The New York Times* and *Cosmopolitan.* She lives in New York City.